ISBN: 9798656503167

90-DAY
Mediterranean Diet
1200-CALORIE

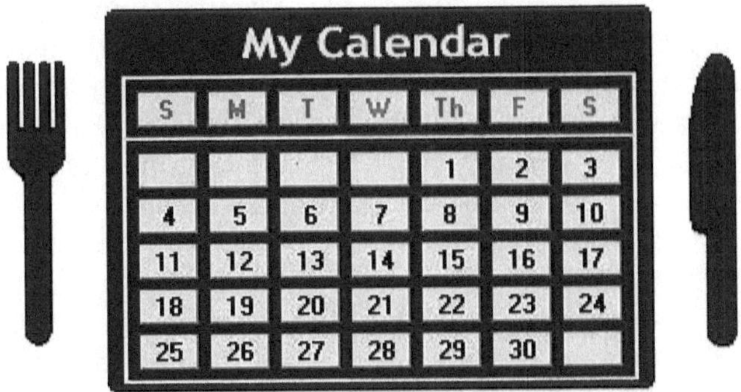

Vincent Antonetti, PhD
Tina Hudson, M.S.

NoPaperPress™

NOTE: At publication, the off-the-shelf foods used in portions of this book were widely available in most supermarkets. But food products come and go. So if there is a frozen entrée or soup selection in this diet that is out of stock, or that's been discontinued, or perhaps that you don't like, or that you forgot to pick up while shopping, please substitute another food that has **approximately** the same caloric value and nutritional content. In this regard, many dieters have found the foods listed in the Appendices at the end of this book to be very helpful.

PREFACE

In 1958, Dr. Ancel Keys, a highly-regarded scientist at the University of Minnesota, started a landmark research project of healthy middle-aged men called The Seven Countries Study[1]. The project lasted decades and included men living in Greece, Italy, Yugoslavia, the Netherlands, Finland, and the United States. His findings supported previous studies that pointed to saturated fats as the cause of the arterial blockages that resulted in heart disease and heart attacks. But he also found that in Mediterranean countries, such as Greece and Italy, heart disease was not as prevalent and caused fewer deaths than in northern Europe and the United States. Dr. Keys was the first to advocate the health implications of a Mediterranean-style diet.

Generally speaking the Mediterranean diet is a way of eating based on the long-established cuisine of the countries bordering the Mediterranean Sea. The diet typically contains lots of vegetables, fruits, whole grain breads, beans, seafood, nut and seeds, olive oil and red wine. Plant-based foods are central to the diet. But moderate amounts of dairy, seafood, poultry and eggs are also important in the Mediterranean Diet. In contrast, red meat is eaten infrequently.

Healthy fats are a mainstay of a Mediterranean diet and are consumed instead of unhealthy saturated and trans fats which contribute to heart disease. Olive oil is the primary source of added fat in a Mediterranean diet. Olive oil is a monounsaturated fat, which has been found to lower total cholesterol and LDL (or "bad") cholesterol levels. Nuts and seeds also contain monounsaturated fat.

Seafood is also important in the Mediterranean diet. Fatty fish such as mackerel, herring, sardines, albacore tuna, salmon and lake trout, all rich in omega-3 fatty acids, a type of polyunsaturated fat that is thought to reduce inflammation in humans. Omega-3 fatty acids also help to decrease triglycerides, reduce blood clotting, and decrease the risk of stroke and congestive heart failure. A typical Mediterranean diet allows red wine - but only in moderation.

Research has shown that the Mediterranean Diet is by far one of the healthiest in the world. It's important to note that the Mediterranean Diet in this book is also a **Reducing Diet** and therefore shows the caloric value of the foods in the diet. In fact, what makes the Mediterranean Diet in this book different is the emphasis on calorie control which is what leads directly to weight loss.

The version of the Mediterranean Diet in this book has been modified slightly to be consistent with American dietary patterns, food preferences and calorie control.

Note that Vince (the primary author) is three-quarters Italian and Tina's mother was of Italian decent. This is the diet we both grew up eating.

Vince Antonetti & Tina Hudson
July 2020

1. Keys, Ancel. "Coronary problems in seven countries." Circulation 41.1 (1970): 186-195.

CONTENTS

1200 CALORIE MEAL PLANS

RECIPIES & DIET TIPS

Day 52 Recipe: Chicken Piccata
Day 53 Recipe: Pasta Primavera (160)
Day 54 Recipe: Grilled Scallops & Polenta
Day 55 Recipe: Hearty Vegetable Soup (162)
Day 56 Recipe: Frozen Chicken Dinner
Day 57 Recipe: Salmon with Mango Salsa (164)
Day 58 Recipe: Grilled Pork Chop with Orange
Day 59 Recipe: Fish Dinner Out (166)
Day 60 Recipe: Chicken Stew over Rice
Day 61 Recipe: Shrimp over Spaghetti (168)
Day 62 Recipe: Beef Burgundy
Day 63 Recipe: Chicken Cutlet (170)
Day 64 Recipe: Turkey Meatloaf
Day 65 Recipe: Frozen Fish Dinner (172)
Day 66 Recipe: Pita Pizza
Day 67 Recipe: Chicken Dinner Out (174)
Day 68 Recipe: Pork Medallions in Lime Sauce
Day 69 Recipe: Healthy Chicken Salad (176)
Day 70 Recipe: Baked Cod
Day 71 Recipe: Chicken Scaloppini (178)
Day 72 Recipe: Fish Dinner Out
Day 73 Recipe: Pasta Pomodoro (180)
Day 74 Recipe: Frozen Chicken Dinner
Day 75 Recipe: Mediterranean Chicken (182)
Day 76 Recipe: Grilled Scallops
Day 77 Recipe: Chicken with Peppers & Rice (184)
Day 78 Recipe: Trout with Lemon & Capers
Day 79 Recipe: Italian Food - Out (186)
Day 80 Recipe: Vegetable Chilli
Day 81 Recipe: Frozen Meat Dinner (188)
Day 82 Recipe: Chicken Salad
Day 83 Recipe: Hearty Lentil Stew (190)
Day 84 Recipe: Turkey Burger
Day 85 Recipe: Lo-Cal Meat Loaf (192)
Day 86 Recipe: Tuna & Bean Salad
Day 87 Recipe: Pasta and Veggies (194)
Day 88 Recipe: Frozen Chicken Dinner
Day 89 Recipe: Fish Stew (196)
Day 90 Recipe: Veal with Mushrooms & Tomato

The Best Weight-Loss Diets

According to the late Dr. Jean Mayer of Harvard University's Department of Nutrition, a really good weight-loss diet must have the following three characteristics:

1) The diet must provide you with an understanding of weight control as well as the knowledge you need to reduce your weight to the desired level.

2) The diet must help you remain healthy while you are losing weight.

3) The diet must lead you to a healthier way of eating and exercising that will, in the long term, help you keep off the weight you have lost.

The Mediterranean weight-loss diet featured in this book is a diet that is not only low calorie and reasonably low in fat, but is also nutritionally balanced. The *90-Day Mediterranean Diet*, however, does not meet all the criteria set forth above. While you will acquire some "dieting insight" and some idea of how much you can eat and still lose weight, you will not get a real understanding of weight control from this book. That's not its purpose. What you will get is a healthy diet – and a diet that if followed will promote weight loss. Think of the *90-Day Mediterranean Diet* as a quick fix, a healthy start that will get you on the right track – but it's not the long-term answer.

Long-term success is about developing both an understanding and a plan that will result in healthier eating and physical activity habits. For a through understanding and the guidance you need to succeed in the long term we recommend you read, *Weight Control - U.S. Edition* by Vincent Antonetti, Ph.D., another NoPaperPress book.

Begin with a Medical Exam

Everyone should at the very least have a medical assessment, or exam, before starting a weight loss diet. Why? You need to make sure your health will allow you to lower your caloric intake and increase your physical activity. The medical checkup may be as simple as a visit to a physician who is familiar with your medical history, or it may be a thorough physical exam. The physician conducting the medical exam should be made aware of and should approve the specific weight loss diet you're planning.

What's in This Book?

This book contains 90 Daily Menus and 90 delicious Recipes.

How Much Weight Will You Lose?

Weight loss occurs when your food energy intake is less than the total energy you expend. This difference in calories is referred to as your calorie deficit. How much weight you lose depends on the magnitude of your calorie deficit. Simple metabolic calculations make a rough estimate possible.

On the 90-Day Mediterranean Diet - 1200 Calorie, most women lose 23 to 33 pounds.

On the 90-Day Mediterranean Diet - 1200 Calorie, most men lose 35 to 45 pounds

Smaller adults, older adults and less active adults might lose a bit less and larger adults, younger adults and more active adults often much more. Exactly how much weight you will lose depends on how much you weigh, your age and your activity level. Again, for the full story see *Weight Control - U.S. Edition* by Vincent Antonetti, Ph.D.

Guidelines for Healthy Eating

Even though most adults can get all the vitamins and minerals they need by merely consuming a variety of nutritious foods (from the fruit group, the vegetable group, the grains group, the meat and beans group, the milk group, and the oils group), many physicians recommend a daily multi-vitamin/mineral supplement – just in case you don't eat the way you should.

Large Salad: One of the dinner mainstays is a "Large Salad." Prepare your "Large Salad" in a bowl with a volume of at least 16 ounces, or 2 cups. First add about 1 cup of either green leaf lettuce, Romaine lettuce or a mesclun mix. Then add, as desired, another cup of other veggies such as broccoli, celery, cucumber, tomato, onion, peppers, spinach, or watercress. This vegetable combination will, on average, total about 40 Calories. You will be eating a "Large Salad" just about every day at dinnertime. Remember that variety is the key to a nutritious diet. So be sure to vary the ingredients of the salad. Top your large salad with two tablespoons of the salad dressing discussed below.

For a "**Small Salad**" use half the ingredients of the preceding large salad and half of the following salad dressing.

Salad Dressing: Mix two tablespoons of extra virgin olive oil (Evoo) with one tablespoon of balsamic vinegar and one tablespoon of water. Add salt, pepper and any Italian herbs to taste. Whisk ingredients together. Shake well. Use half of the dressing on your large salad. Save the remainder in your fridge.

Your "Large Salad" with salad dressing will cost you roughly 150 Calories but will be packed with lots of health-giving vitamins, minerals and fiber. The "Small Salad" contains about 75 Calories.

Homemade Cooking Spray: Simply combine one part olive oil with one part water into a spray bottle. Shake well and spray! Cheap, low calorie and effective.

Soup: See Appendix C page 205 for a list of the soup permitted on this diet. To improve the taste of a canned soup, add a teaspoon of grated cheese before heating in a microwave oven. After heating, add ½ teaspoon of olive oil. Stir and serve. These additions total about 30 Calories but really enhance the taste.

About Bread: First understand that bread, more specifically whole-grain breads, are good sources of complex carbohydrates and dietary fiber, as well as several B vitamins (thiamin, riboflavin, niacin, and foliate), vitamin E, and minerals (iron, magnesium and selenium). In recent years, however, sliced bread loaves have gotten larger, as have the bread slices inside these loaves. Just a few years ago the standard slice of bread contained about 65 to 70 Calories – now most are 100 plus Calories.

The *90-Day Mediterranean Diet* requires whole-grain bread at 65 to 70 Calories per slice for breakfast toast. Quite a few bakers sell thin sliced or "light" sliced bread. The difficult part is finding a whole grain thin sliced or "light" bread (with about 70 Calories per slice). Whatever the brand, make sure the first word in the Ingredients list is "whole." "Pepperidge Farm Small Slice 100% Whole Wheat" is a good breakfast choice. It's whole grain, has 70 Calories per slice and it tastes good too.

For dinner find a good loaf of **Italian or French bread** and use about one ounce (80 Calories). <u>Hint</u>: Get the weight of the loaf from a label, or weigh it on a scale in the produce section of the store. Then estimate how many one ounce servings the loaf contains and slice accordingly.

Exchanging Foods

If there is a food listed in the *90-Day Mediterranean Diet* that you don't like, or perhaps that you forgot to pick up while shopping, you probably can exchange or substitute another food in its place – a technique used by dieticians. Exchanging a food listed in a diet for another food with approximately equal caloric value and nutritional content is the foundation of a successful long-term diet. Substitution possibilities are almost endless but have to be done carefully.

The easiest substitutions are those within the same food group, such as exchanging one vegetable variety for another, or a glass of milk for a cup of yogurt. More sophisticated exchanges cross food groups, for instance replacing 3½ ounces of turkey with a tablespoon of peanut butter spread on a piece of whole wheat bread. Both foods are complete protein and both contain about 175 Calories.

Refer to a good online calorie table. With some understanding and experience, you can use this table to help you substitute foods called for in the *Mediterranean Diet* with equal calorie foods from the same food group.

Breakfast: You may substitute any cereal for any other wholesome cereal. For example, if you're not crazy about having Shredded Wheat for breakfast, substitute Wheat Chex or Cheerios, etc. If you don't like the soft-boiled egg called for on Day 9, make yourself a scrambled egg instead. And if Cantaloupe is on the menu but is not in season, replace the cantaloupe with a half cup of orange juice.

Snacks: Again, where yogurt is specified you may substitute a 6-ounce glass of skim milk, but to maintain a nutritionally balanced diet keep this snack a dairy selection. Similarly, when fruit is on the agenda, you may select another type of fruit but do not stray from the fruit group. Nuts and popcorn can be interchanged at will. (Incidentally, you should buy a hot-air popper. They make great popcorn – which is high in fiber and makes a tasty and nutritious snack.)

Two Nights Off

Everyone deserves a break from the grind of preparing dinner after coming home from work. So the *90-Day Mediterranean Diet* gives you two days off per week! Notice that one night a week the diet calls for a frozen dinner and on a second night during the week you're encouraged to eat out. There are, however, some rules and caveats involved and these are covered in the next two sections.

Frozen Dinners

In general, a frozen dinner should not be a meal in itself. Make sure you add a salad, fruit, bread etc. The frozen dinner you choose should come with at least one cup of cooked vegetables. If your frozen dinner doesn't measure up, add your own frozen, fresh or canned vegetables. And look for dinners with no more than 800 mg of sodium. In addition, make sure the dinner you choose has no more than 30 percent of the daily value for total fat. Appendix A page 198 lists almost 150 frozen dinner entrees.

And on the days when a frozen dinner is specified, you will also be given a calorie goal for the frozen dinner. For example, Day 5 calls for frozen fish dinner with a maximum allowable 300 Calories. If you choose a frozen fish dinner that contains less than 300 Calories, you may spend the unused calories any way you wish.

Moreover, on those nights when you just don't have the energy or time to cook, you can always substitute a frozen dinner for the entree listed in the meal plan. For example, Day 1 calls for Chicken with Peppers and Onions for dinner. The total calorie count for dinner is 500. In place of the Day 1 calls for Chicken with Peppers and Onions, any combination of a frozen chicken dinner and side dishes (salads, etc) with a total calorie content close to 500 would be an acceptable, albeit not as tasty, an alternative.

Eating Out

You may eat out once a week. When you're on a diet, however, eating in a restaurant can be a challenge, because most restaurant portions are huge, and can easily total more than 1,000 Calories. On the *90-Day Mediterranean Diet*, a dinner type (i.e., fish, chicken, etc) and a calorie target is specified. For example Day 7 of the 1500 Calorie diet specifies a chicken dinner and allows you 630 Calories.

First, you need to choose a restaurant where you have a fighting chance to achieve your calorie goal. Next, order simple, such as broiled chicken breast with steamed vegetables and brown rice. Tell the waiter you want no sauce, no gravy, nothing added. Then, knowing your calorie objective, and that most fish and chicken are about 50 Calories per ounce, most steamed vegetable servings average about 50 Calories per cup, and rice is about 100 Calories per ½ cup, decide how much to eat – and take the remainder home. If fresh fruit is not an option, pass on dessert and have the evening snack specified in the meal plan for that day.

Mediterranean Diet Info

As mentioned previously, the 1200 Calorie 90-Day Diet starts on page 17. There is a detailed meal plan for each of the 90 days. Associated with each day is a "Recipe of the Day" and a "Diet Tip of the Day."

After you complete the 90th day on the diet, if you still want to lose more weight a good alternative is to repeat the diet by starting over at Day1.

Important Notes

1) Coffee may be decaf or regular. If desired, skim milk and a sugar substitute may be added to coffee or tea.

2) Fried eggs or scrambled eggs should be cooked in a pan coated with a non-stick cooking spray (see page 11). Hard-boiled eggs may be substituted for fried, scrambled or soft-boiled eggs.

3) Cereals should be whole grain and unsweetened. At the top of the list are Old-fashioned Oatmeal, Wheatena and Shredded Wheat. Among other reasonably healthy choices are Cheerios, Wheat Chex, Wheaties, some Kashi cereals and Farina. When blueberries are in season, you may add blueberries instead of raisins to your cereal. (Substitution ratio = 2 blueberries per raisin.)

4) Bread may be either plain or toasted whole grain, such as whole wheat, whole rye or pumpernickel. Look for whole grain varieties that contain 70 Calories per slice. If desired, bread may be topped with a home-made low-calorie olive oil spray. NO BUTTER!

5) When soup is specified, have only one serving (8 ounces) unless otherwise noted. (Most caned soups usually contain about two servings.)

6) Use freely as desired: clear unsweetened coffee, clear unsweetened tea, water, seltzer water and any diet soda, clear soups without fat, bouillon, and seasonings such as mustard, cinnamon, dill, herbs, red and black pepper, curry, vinegar, and lemon juice and lemon sections.

7) Use only lean cuts of meat trimmed of all visible fat. Poultry should be limited to chicken or turkey breasts (white meat only and skinless).

8) When canned tuna or salmon is specified, use only fish packed in water.

9) When the diet calls for turkey bacon, make sure the brand you buy has no more than 35 Calories per slice.

10) An unlimited amount of salad may be eaten, but the salad dressing should be as specified on page 11.

11) Use freely as desired: clear unsweetened coffee, clear unsweetened tea, water, seltzer, any diet soda, clear soups without fat, bouillon, and seasonings such as mustard, cinnamon, dill, herbs, red and black pepper, curry, vinegar, lemon juice and sections, and dill and sour pickles.

12) If it's more convenient, any food item may be moved to any part of the day and combined with any meal or snack.

13) If you cannot find the exact item called for in the diet (because it's out of stock or discontinued), substitute a comparable food (of the same type and close caloric value).

14) Although it's recommended that you follow the diet days as outlined, it's fine to occasionally pick and choose the days you prefer. (

1200 CALORIE DAILY MENUS

Day 1 – 1200 Calorie Meal Plan

BREAKFAST	Calories	Totals
Grapefruit (½)	75	
Scrambled egg (page 14)	80	
Whole-grain toast (1 slice) (page 11)	65	
Coffee (page 14)	10	230 Cal
SNACK		
Coffee or tea	10	10 Cal
LUNCH		
Salad – 3 oz canned salmon, 1 tsp Evoo, onions & celery	200	
Lettuce & tomato wedges	20	
Italian or French bread (1 slice) (page 14)	80	
Water	0	300 Cal
SNACK		
Greek Yogurt (6 oz, nonfat, any flavor)*	90	90 Cal
DINNER		
Chicken w Peppers & Onions (Day 1 Recipe p. 108)	250	
Sautéed red peppers with onions	70	
Green beans (steamed) & mashed cauliflower	45	
Large salad with 2 Tbsp dressing (page 10)	150	
Water	0	515 Cal
SNACK		
Fresh fruit in season (apple, plum, etc)	70	70 Cal
* Such as, Dannon Lite & Fit. (Buy 32 oz container & use 6 oz.)		1215 Cal

Day 2 – 1200 Calorie Meal Plan

BREAKFAST	Calories	Totals
Fresh or frozen strawberries (½ cup)	25	
French toasted English Muffin (Day 2 Recipe p 109)	270	
Light syrup (1 Tbsp)	30	
Coffee	10	335 Cal
SNACK		
Coffee or tea	10	10 Cal
LUNCH		
Salad (3 oz tuna, 1 tsp Evoo, onions & celery)	175	
Lettuce & tomato wedges	20	
Italian or French bread (1 slice) (page 14)	80	
Hot or iced tea	10	285 Cal
SNACK		
Greek Yogurt (6 oz, nonfat, any flavor)	90	
Coffee or tea	10	100 Cal
DINNER		
Broiled veal chop (4 oz lean)	200	
Broccoli (½ cup steamed)	25	
Large salad with 2 Tbsp dressing (page 10)	150	
Glass wine (red or white) (4 oz)	100	395 Cal
SNACK		
Fresh fruit in season (apple, peach, etc)	70	70 Cal
		1205 Cal

Day 3 – 1200 Calorie Meal Plan

BREAKFAST	Calories	Totals
Orange juice (½ cup)	50	
Wheaties (¾ cup) + ½ cup skim milk + ½ banana	190	
Coffee	10	250 Cal
SNACK		
Fresh fruit in season (apple, peach, etc)	70	70 Cal
LUNCH		
Soup # 1 (Appendix C - page 205)*	110	
Turkey breast (1 oz) on 1 slice bread (½ sandwich)	105	
Lettuce & tomato slices	20	
Hot or ice tea	10	245 Cal
* 30 calories added to account for flavor enhancement.		
SNACK		
Coffee or tea	10	10 Cal
DINNER		
Baked Herb-Crusted Cod (Day 3 Recipe page 110)	230	
Spinach (½ cup) steamed with garlic & drizzled Evoo	100	
Asparagus (7 spear cooked & drained)	20	
Italian or French bread (1 slice)	80	
Glass wine (red or white) (4 oz)	100	
Water	0	530 Cal
SNACK		
Fiber One Chocolate Fudge Brownie	90	
Coffee or tea	10	100 Cal
		1200 Cal

Day 4 – 1200 Calorie Meal Plan

BREAKFAST	Calories	Totals
Grapefruit (½)	**75**	
Cheerios (1 cup) + ½ cup skim milk + about 15 raisins*	**180**	
Coffee	**10**	**265 Cal**
SNACK		
Coffee or tea	**10**	**10 Cal**
LUNCH		
Subway 6" Sandwich (Roast Beef, Cheese + veggies)**	**245**	
Large salad with 2 Tbsp dressing (page 10)	**150**	
Water	**0**	**395 Cal**
** On 6" half wheat roll.		
SNACK		
Fresh fruit in season (peach, plum, etc)	**70**	**70 Cal**
DINNER		
Pasta and Veggies (Day 4 Recipe - page 111)	**460**	
Water	**0**	**460 Cal**
SNACK		
Coffee or tea	**10**	**10 Cal**
* See page 14 re substituting blueberries for raisins.		**1210 Cal**

Day 5 – 1200 Calorie Meal Plan

BREAKFAST	Calories	Totals
Cantaloupe (½ medium)	50	
Fried egg	80	
Toasted raisin bread (1 slice)	75	
Coffee	10	215 Cal
SNACK		
Coffee or tea	10	10 Cal
LUNCH		
Soup #5 (Appendix C - page 205)	140	
Italian or French bread (1 slice)	80	
Lettuce and sliced tomato with 1 Tbsp dressing	85	
Hot or iced tea	10	315 Cal
* 30 calories added to account for flavor enhancement.		
SNACK		
Greek Yogurt (6 oz, nonfat, any flavor)	90	90 Cal
DINNER		
Frozen fish dinner (Day 5 Recipe - page 112)	340	
Large salad with 2 Tbsp dressing	150	
Water	0	490 Cal
SNACK		
One small cookie*	80	
Coffee or tea	10	90 Cal
* Oatmeal, ginger snap, sugar, etc - check calories!		1210 Cal

Day 6 – 1200 Calorie Meal Plan

BREAKFAST	Calories	Totals
Tomato juice (½ cup)	20	
Shredded Wheat (1 cup) + ½ cup skim milk + ½ banana	265	
Coffee	10	295 Cal
SNACK		
Coffee or tea	10	10 Cal
LUNCH		
Ham (2 oz) with mustard on 2 slices rye bread	290	
Lettuce	10	
Hot or iced tea	10	310 Cal
SNACK		
Fresh fruit in season (pear, plum, etc)	70	70 Cal
DINNER		
Pizza (Day 6 Recipe - page 113)	350	
Large salad with 2 Tbsp dressing	150	
Water or diet soda	0	490 Cal
SNACK		
Coffee or tea	10	10 Cal
		1185 Cal

Day 7 – 1200 Calorie Meal Plan

BREAKFAST	Calories	Totals
Cantaloupe (½ medium)	50	
Oatmeal (½ cup dry) + ½ cup skim milk + about 15 raisins	220	
Coffee	10	280 Cal
SNACK		
Coffee or tea	10	10 Cal
LUNCH		
Grilled cheese sandwich (2 slices 2% cheese)	230	
Lettuce and sliced tomato	20	
Water	0	250 Cal
SNACK		
Carrot sticks + ¼ cup low-fat cottage cheese & chives	60	60 Cal
DINNER		
Eat Out – Chicken dinner (Day 7 Recipe - page 116)	480	
Glass wine (red or white) (4 oz)	100	580 Cal
SNACK		
Coffee or tea	10	10 Cal
		1190 Cal

Day 8 – 1200 Calorie Meal Plan

BREAKFAST	Calories	Totals
Cantaloupe (½ medium)	50	
Wheaties (¾ cup) + ½ cup skim milk + ½ banana	190	
Coffee	10	250 Cal
SNACK		
Coffee or tea	10	10 Cal
LUNCH		
Soup #2 (Appendix C - page 205)*	120	
Turkey (1 oz) on 1 slice of rye bread (½ sandwich)	115	
Lettuce & tomato slices	20	
Hot or iced tea	10	265 Cal
* 30 calories added to account for flavor enhancement.		
SNACK		
Small bunch of grapes	65	65 Cal
DINNER		
Baked salmon with salsa (Day 8 Recipe - page 115)	215	
Summer squash, zucchini and tomatoes	60	
Brown rice (½ cup)	100	
Large salad with 2 Tbsp dressing	150	
Water with lemon wedge	15	540 Cal
SNACK		
Fresh fruit in season (apple, plum, etc)	70	70 Cal
		1200 Cal

Day 9 – 1200 Calorie Meal Plan

BREAKFAST	Calories	Totals
Orange juice (½ cup)	50	
Soft-boiled egg	80	
Whole-grain toast (1 slice)	65	
Coffee	10	205 Cal
SNACK		
Coffee or tea	10	10 Cal
LUNCH		
Salad (3 oz tuna, 1 tsp Evoo, onions & celery)	175	
Lettuce & tomato wedges	20	
Rye bread (1 slice)	65	
Fresh fruit in season (pear, peach, etc)	70	
Water or diet soda	0	330 Cal
SNACK		
Greek Yogurt (6 oz, nonfat, any flavor)	90	
Coffee or tea	10	100 Cal
DINNER		
Veggie burger – (1 patty) (Day 9 Recipe - page 116)	100	
Low-fat cheddar cheese (1 thin slice)	50	
Seeded hamburger roll + Beets (3 small)	185	
Large salad with 2 Tbsp dressing	150	
Water	0	475 Cal
SNACK		
One small cookie	80	
Coffee or tea	10	90 Cal
		1210 Cal

Day 10 – 1200 Calorie Meal Plan

BREAKFAST	Calories	Totals
Orange juice (½ cup)	50	
Wild blueberry pancakes (Day 10 Recipe - page 117)	190	
Light syrup (1½ Tbsp)	45	
Coffee	10	295 Cal
SNACK		
Coffee or tea	10	10 Cal
LUNCH		
Peanut butter (2 Tbsp) on 2 slices whole-grain bread	330	
Skim milk (4 oz)	45	
Fresh fruit in season (apple, plum, etc)	70	445 Cal
SNACK		
Coffee or tea	10	10 Cal
DINNER		
Broiled pork chop (about ½" thick & trimmed of fat)	260	
Green peas (½ cup)	55	
Tomato & cucumbers salad with 1 Tbsp dressing	105	
Water with lemon wedge	10	430Cal
SNACK		
Coffee or tea	10	10 Cal
		1200 Cal

Day 11 – 1200 Calorie Meal Plan

BREAKFAST	Calories	Totals
Fresh sliced orange	75	
Cheerios (1 cup) + ½ cup skim milk + about 15 raisins	190	
Coffee	10	275 Cal
SNACK		
Fresh fruit in season (apple, plum, etc)	70	70 Cal
LUNCH		
Subway 6" Sandwich (Ham, Cheese + veggies)	260	
Water or diet soda	0	260 Cal
SNACK		
Handful unsalted mixed nuts	100	100 Cal
DINNER		
Grilled chicken sausage (2 links about 2½ oz per link)	180	
Artichoke-bean salad (Day 11 Recipe - page 118)	190	
Green beans - steamed	25	
Glass of wine (4 oz)	100	495 Cal
SNACK		
Coffee or tea	10	10 Cal
		1210 Cal

Day 12 – 1200 Calorie Meal Plan

BREAKFAST	Calories	Totals
Grapefruit (½)	75	
Scrambled egg	80	
Whole-grain toast (1 slice)	65	
Coffee	10	230 Cal
SNACK		
Coffee or tea	10	10 Cal
LUNCH		
Soup #4 (Appendix C - page 205)	140	
Tomato slices, ¼ cup chopped fresh basil + ½ tsp Evoo	40	
Whole-grain bread (1 slice)	65	
Hot or iced tea	10	265 Cal
* 30 calories added to account for flavor enhancement.		
SNACK		
Greek Yogurt (6 oz, nonfat, any flavor)	90	
Coffee or tea	10	100 Cal
DINNER		
Eat Out – Fish dinner (Day 12 Recipe page 119)	495	
Glass of wine (4 oz)	100	595 Cal
SNACK		
Coffee or tea	10	10 Cal
		1210 Cal

Day 13 – 1200 Calorie Meal Plan

BREAKFAST	Calories	Totals
Orange juice (½ cup)	50	
Shredded Wheat (1 cup) + ½ cup skim milk + ½ banana	260	
Coffee	10	320 Cal
SNACK		
Coffee or tea	10	10 Cal
LUNCH		
Turkey frank (2 oz) with mustard & relish	150	
Hot dog bun	125	
Water or diet soda	0	275 Cal
SNACK		
Fresh fruit in season (pear, plum, etc)	70	70 Cal
DINNER		
Pasta with Marinara sauce (Day 13 Recipe - p. 120)	225	
Large salad with 2 Tbsp dressing	150	
Italian or French bread (1 slice)	80	
Water	0	455 Cal
SNACK		
Fiber One Chocolate Fudge Brownie	90	90 Cal
		1220 Cal

Day 14 – 1200 Calorie Meal Plan

BREAKFAST	Calories	Totals
Cantaloupe (½ medium)	50	
Oatena cereal mix (Day 14 Recipe - page 121)	310	
Coffee	10	370 Cal
SNACK		
Coffee or tea	10	10 Cal
LUNCH		
Grilled Swiss cheese sandwich (2 oz low-fat cheese)	310	
Diet soda or water	0	310 Cal
SNACK		
Small bunch of grapes	65	65 Cal
DINNER		
Frozen chicken dinner (Day 28 Recipe - page 135)	300	
Small salad with 1 Tbsp dressing	75	
Water	0	375 Cal
SNACK		
Greek Yogurt (6 oz, nonfat, any flavor)	90	90 Cal
		1220 Cal

Day 15 – 1200 Calorie Meal Plan

BREAKFAST	Calories	Totals
Fresh or frozen strawberries (1 cup)	50	
French toast (2 slices whole-grain bread & 1 egg)	250	
Light syrup (1 Tbsp)	30	
Coffee	10	340 Cal
SNACK		
Coffee or tea	10	10 Cal
LUNCH		
Salad (3 oz tuna, 1 tsp Evoo, onions & celery)	175	
Lettuce & tomato wedges	20	
Rye bread (1 slice)	65	
Coffee or tea	10	270 Cal
SNACK		
Greek Yogurt (6 oz, nonfat, any flavor)	90	
Coffee or tea	10	100 Cal
DINNER		
London broil (Day 15 Recipe - page 122)	320	
Brown rice (½ cup)	100	
Broccoli (1 cup steamed)	50	
Water	0	470 Cal
SNACK		
Coffee or tea	10	10 Cal
		1200 Cal

Day 16 – 1200 Calorie Meal Plan

BREAKFAST	Calories	Totals
Orange juice (½ cup)	50	
Wheat Chex (¾ cup) + ½ cup skim milk + ½ banana	250	
Coffee	10	310 Cal
SNACK		
Coffee or tea	10	10 Cal
LUNCH		
Subway 6" Sandwich (Roast Beef, Cheese + veggies)	245	
Diet soda or water	0	245 Cal
SNACK		
Fresh fruit in season (apple, peach, etc)	70	
Coffee or tea	10	80 Cal
DINNER		
Baked red snapper (Day 16 Recipe - page 123)	215	
Wild rice mix	160	
Green beans & tomato	75	
Water with lemon section	15	465 Cal
SNACK		
Greek Yogurt (6 oz, nonfat, any flavor)	90	
Coffee or tea	10	100 Cal
		1200 Cal

Day 17 – 1200 Calorie Meal Plan

BREAKFAST	Calories	Totals
Cantaloupe (½ medium)	50	
Fried egg	80	
Turkey bacon (1 slice)	35	
Toasted raisin bread (1 slice)	75	
Coffee	10	250 Cal
SNACK		
Coffee or tea	10	10 Cal
LUNCH		
Soup #7 (Appendix C - page 205)	160	
Lettuce & tomato sandwich with Tbsp light mayo	170	
Cucumber slices and carrot & celery sticks	15	
Hot or iced tea	10	355 Cal
SNACK		
Greek Yogurt (6 oz, nonfat, any flavor)	90	90 Cal
DINNER		
Cajun chicken salad (Day 17 Recipe - page 124)	330	
Whole-grain bread (1 slice)	65	
Fresh fruit in season (pear, plum, etc)	70	
Water with lemon section	10	475 Cal
SNACK		
Coffee or tea	10	10 Cal
		1190 Cal

Day 18 – 1200 Calorie Meal Plan

BREAKFAST	Calories	Totals
Grapefruit (½)	75	
Cheerios (1 cup) + ½ cup skim milk + about 15 raisins	190	
Coffee	10	275 Cal
SNACK		
Coffee or tea	10	10 Cal
LUNCH		
Cottage cheese (1 cup low fat)	180	
Small salad with 1 Tbsp low-cal dressing (page 10)	75	
Hot or iced tea	10	265 Cal
SNACK		
Handful unsalted mixed nuts	100	
Coffee or tea	10	110 Cal
DINNER		
Grilled swordfish (Day 18 Recipe - page 125)	250	
Grilled potatoes	100	
Grilled cherry tomatoes	40	
Spinach (½ cup) steamed with garlic & drizzled Evoo	50	
Glass of wine (4 oz)	100	540 Cal
SNACK		
Coffee or tea	10	10 Cal
		1210 Cal

Day 19 – 1200 Calorie Meal Plan

BREAKFAST	Calories	Totals
Grapefruit (½)	75	
Scrambled egg	80	
Whole-grain toast (1 slice)	65	
Coffee	10	230 Cal
SNACK		
Coffee or tea	10	10 Cal
LUNCH		
Soup #9 (Appendix C - page 205)	180	
Turkey (1 oz) on 1 slice of rye bread (½ sandwich)	115	
Hot or iced tea	10	305 Cal
SNACK		
Coffee or tea	10	10 Cal
DINNER		
Eat Out – Italian food (Day 19 Recipe - page 126)	540	
Glass of wine (4 oz)	100	640 Cal
SNACK		
Coffee or tea	10	10 Cal
		1205 Cal

Day 20 – 1200 Calorie Meal Plan

BREAKFAST	Calories	Totals
Tomato juice (½ cup)	20	
Shredded Wheat (1 cup) + ½ cup skim milk	210	
Coffee	10	240 Cal
SNACK		
Handful unsalted mixed nuts	100	100 Cal
LUNCH		
Left over Italian food from Day 19	260	
Hot or iced tea	10	270 Cal
SNACK		
Greek Yogurt (6 oz, nonfat, any flavor)	90	90 Cal
DINNER		
Spaghetti alla Puttanesca (Day 20 Recipe - page 127)	345	
Large salad with 2 Tbsp dressing	150	
Water	0	495 Cal
SNACK		
Coffee or tea	10	10 Cal
		1205 Cal

Day 21 – 1200 Calorie Meal Plan

BREAKFAST	Calories	Totals
Cantaloupe (½ medium)	50	
Oatmeal (½ cup dry) + ½ cup skim milk + about 15 raisins	220	
Coffee	10	280 Cal
SNACK		
Coffee or tea	10	10 Cal
LUNCH		
Turkey breast (2 oz) sandwich	235	
Lettuce & tomato with Tbsp light mayo	35	
Fresh fruit in season (apple, plum, etc)	70	
Water	0	340 Cal
SNACK		
Coffee or tea	10	10 Cal
DINNER		
Frozen meat dinner (Day 21 Recipe - page 128)	300	
Large salad with 2 Tbsp dressing	150	
Glass of wine (4 oz)	100	550 Cal
SNACK		
Coffee or tea	10	10 Cal
		1200 Cal

Day 22 – 1200 Calorie Meal Plan

BREAKFAST	Calories	Totals
Fresh or frozen strawberries (1 cup)	25	
French toasted English Muffin (Day 2 Recipe p.109)	270	
Light syrup (1 Tbsp)	30	
Coffee	10	335 Cal
SNACK		
Coffee or tea	10	10 Cal
LUNCH		
Salad (3 oz tuna, 1 tsp Evoo, onions & celery)	175	
Lettuce & tomato wedges	20	
Italian or French bread (1 slice)	80	
Hot or iced tea	10	285 Cal
SNACK		
Coffee or tea	10	10 Cal
DINNER		
Shrimp & spinach salad (Day 22 Recipe - page 129)	310	
Italian or French bread (1 slice)	80	
Large salad with 2 Tbsp dressing	150	
Water	0	540 Cal
SNACK		
Coffee or tea	10	10 Cal
		1190 Cal

Day 23 – 1200 Calorie Meal Plan

BREAKFAST	Calories	Totals
Cantaloupe (½ medium)	50	
Wheaties (¾ cup) + ½ cup skim milk + ½ banana	190	
Whole-grain toast (1 slice)	65	
Coffee	10	315 Cal
SNACK		
Coffee or tea	10	10 Cal
LUNCH		
Ham (2 oz) with mustard on 2 slices rye bread	290	
Lettuce & tomato wedges	20	
Water or diet soda	0	310 Cal
SNACK		
Handful unsalted mixed nuts	100	
Coffee or tea	10	110 Cal
DINNER		
Beans & greens salad (Day 23 Recipe - page 130)	260	
Baked potato (medium)	100	
Water	0	360 Cal
SNACK		
Fresh fruit in season (apple, peach, etc)	70	70 Cal
		1185 Cal

Day 24 – 1200 Calorie Meal Plan

BREAKFAST	Calories	Totals
Fresh orange sliced	75	
Soft-boiled egg	80	
Whole-grain toast (1 slice)	65	
Coffee	10	230 Cal
SNACK		
Greek Yogurt (6 oz, nonfat, any flavor)	90	90 Cal
LUNCH		
Salad – 3 oz salmon, 1 tsp Evoo, onions & celery	200	
Lettuce & tomato wedges	20	
Rye bread (1 slice)	65	
Coffee or tea	10	295 Cal
SNACK		
Coffee or tea	10	10 Cal
DINNER		
Chicken breast – broiled (5 oz)	240	
Four bean plus salad (½ cup) (Day 24 Recipe p 131)	135	
Large salad with 2 Tbsp dressing	150	
Water	0	525 Cal
SNACK		
Fresh fruit in season (pear, plum, etc)	70	70 Cal
		1220 Cal

Day 25 – 1200 Calorie Meal Plan

BREAKFAST	Calories	Totals
Grapefruit (½)	75	
Cheerios (1 cup) + ½ cup skim milk + about 15 raisins	190	
Coffee	10	275 Cal
SNACK		
Coffee or tea	10	10 Cal
LUNCH		
Subway 6" Sandwich (Ham, Cheese + veggies)	260	
Diet soda or water	0	260 Cal
SNACK		
Fresh fruit in season (peach, plum, etc)	70	
Coffee or tea	10	80 Cal
DINNER		
Hanger steak (Day 25 Recipe - page 132)	320	
Roasted potatoes (Day 25 Recipe)	120	
Cherry tomatoes (Day 25 Recipe)	20	
Steamed spinach (½ cup)	25	
Glass of wine (4 oz)	100	585 Cal
SNACK		
Coffee or tea	10	10 Cal
		1220 Cal

Day 26 – 1200 Calorie Meal Plan

BREAKFAST	Calories	Totals
Cantaloupe (½ medium)	50	
Fried egg	80	
Toasted whole-grain bread (1 slice)	65	
Coffee	10	205 Cal
SNACK		
Greek Yogurt (6 oz, nonfat, any flavor)	90	
Coffee or tea	10	100 Cal
LUNCH		
Soup #10 (Appendix C - page 205)	200	
Italian or French bread (1 slice)	80	
Lettuce & tomato slices	20	
Hot or iced tea	10	310 Cal
SNACK		
Fresh fruit in season (apple, plum, etc)	70	
Coffee or tea	10	80 Cal
DINNER		
Grilled scallops (Day 26 Recipe - page 133)	210	
Grilled polenta (Day 26 Recipe)	125	
Mushroom-steamed green beans-red onion	45	
Grilled asparagus	10	
Water	0	390 Cal
SNACK		
Popcorn Mini Bag	110	
Coffee or tea	10	120 Cal
		1205 Cal

Day 27 – 1200 Calorie Meal Plan

BREAKFAST	Calories	Totals
Cantaloupe (½ medium)	50	
Oatmeal (½ cup dry) + ½ cup skim milk + 15 raisins	220	
Coffee	10	280 Cal
SNACK		
Fresh fruit in season (pear, plum, etc)	70	70 Cal
LUNCH		
Two servings (1 cup) left over Day 24 bean salad	270	
Italian or French bread (1 slice)	80	
Lettuce & tomato slices	20	
Water	0	370 Cal
SNACK		
Coffee or tea	10	10 Cal
DINNER		
Fettuccine (Day 27 Recipe - page 134)	290	
Small salad with 1 Tbsp dressing (page 10)	75	
Glass of wine (4 oz)	100	465 Cal
SNACK		
Coffee or tea	10	10 Cal
		1205 Cal

Day 28 – 1200 Calorie Meal Plan

BREAKFAST	Calories	Totals
Tomato juice (½ cup)	20	
Shredded Wheat (1 cup) + ½ cup skim milk + ½ banana	260	
Coffee	10	290 Cal
SNACK		
Coffee or tea	10	10 Cal
LUNCH		
Roast beef sandwich (2 oz) on whole-grain bread	295	
Lettuce	0	
Fresh fruit in season (peach, plum, etc)	70	
Hot or iced tea	10	375 Cal
SNACK		
Handful unsalted mixed nuts	100	
Coffee or tea	10	110 Cal
DINNER		
Frozen chicken dinner (Day 28 Recipe - page 135)	300	
Large salad with 2 Tbsp dressing	150	
Water	0	435 Cal
SNACK		
Coffee or tea	10	10 Cal
		1220 Cal

Day 29 – 1200 Calorie Meal Plan

BREAKFAST	Calories	Totals
Orange juice (½ cup)	50	
Wild blueberry pancakes (Day 10 Recipe - page 117)	190	
Turkey bacon (1 slice)	35	
Light syrup (1 Tbsp)	30	
Coffee	10	315 Cal
SNACK		
Greek Yogurt (6 oz, nonfat, any flavor)	90	
Coffee or tea	10	100 Cal
LUNCH		
Salad (3 oz tuna, 1 tsp Evoo, onions & celery)	175	
Lettuce & tomato wedges	20	
Italian or French bread	80	
Hot or ice tea	10	285 Cal
SNACK		
Coffee or tea	10	10 Cal
DINNER		
Barbequed shrimp (Day 29 Recipe - page 136)	160	
Corn on the cob (medium)	100	
Steamed broccoli (1 cup equivalent)	50	
Glass of wine (4 oz)	100	410 Cal
SNACK		
Fresh fruit in season (apple, peach, etc)	70	70 Cal
		1190 Cal

Day 30 – 1200 Calorie Meal Plan

BREAKFAST	Calories	Totals
Fresh orange sliced	75	
Wheat Chex (¾ cup) + ½ cup skim milk + ½ banana	250	
Coffee	10	335 Cal
SNACK		
Coffee or tea	10	10 Cal
LUNCH		
Soup #8 (Appendix C - page 205)	170	
Italian or French bread (1 slice)	80	
Raw zucchini slices, celery & carrot sticks	20	
Hot or iced tea	10	280 Cal
SNACK		
Coffee or tea	10	10 Cal
DINNER		
Pasta e Fagioli (Day 30 Recipe - page 137)	300	
Small salad with 1 Tbsp dressing	75	
Italian or French bread (1 slice)	80	
Glass of wine (4 oz)	100	555 Cal
SNACK		
Coffee or tea	10	10 Cal
		1200 Cal

Day 31 – 1200 Calorie Meal Plan

BREAKFAST	Calories	Totals
Tomato juice (½ cup)	20	
Wheaties (¾ cup) + ½ cup skim milk	140	
Coffee	10	170 Cal
SNACK		
Coffee or tea	10	10 Cal
LUNCH		
Ham (2 oz) with mustard on 2 slices rye bread	300	
Water	0	300 Cal
SNACK		
Fresh fruit in season (apple, plum, etc)	70	70 Cal
DINNER		
Baked Sea Bass (Day 31 Recipe - page 138)	395	
Small salad with 1 Tbsp dressing	75	
Italian or French bread (1 slice)	80	
Glass of wine (4 oz)	100	650 Cal
SNACK		
Coffee or tea	10	10 Cal
		1210 Cal

Day 32 – 1200 Calorie Meal Plan

BREAKFAST	Calories	Totals
Tomato juice (½ cup)	20	
Cheerios (1 cup) + ½ cup skim milk + about 15 raisins	190	
Coffee	10	220 Cal
SNACK		
Handful unsalted mixed nuts	100	100 Cal
LUNCH		
Soup #2 (Appendix C - page 205)	120	
Italian or French bread (1 slice)	80	
Raw zucchini slices, celery and carrot sticks	20	
Water	0	220 Cal
SNACK		
Fresh fruit in season (apple, plum, etc)	70	70 Cal
DINNER		
Turkey tenders & veggies (Day 32 Recipe - page 139)	350	
Spinach (½ cup steamed & drizzled w 1 tsp Evoo)	70	
Small salad with 1 Tbsp dressing	75	
Glass of wine (4 oz)	100	595 Cal
SNACK		
Coffee or tea	10	10 Cal
		1215 Cal

Day 33 – 1200 Calorie Meal Plan

BREAKFAST	Calories	Totals
Cantaloupe (½ medium)	50	
Fried egg	80	
Toasted raisin bread (1 slice)	75	
Coffee	10	215 Cal
SNACK		
Greek Yogurt (6 oz, nonfat, any flavor)	90	90 Cal
LUNCH		
Subway 6" (Turkey Breast, Cheese + veggies)	230	
Fresh fruit in season (apple, plum, etc)	70	
Water	0	300 Cal
SNACK		
Coffee or tea	10	10 Cal
DINNER		
Frozen fish dinner (Day 33 Recipe - page 140)	340	
Small salad with 1 Tbsp dressing	75	
Glass of wine (4 oz)	100	
Water	0	515 Cal
SNACK		
Small cookie	80	
Coffee or tea	10	90 Cal
		1220 Cal

Day 34 – 1200 Calorie Meal Plan

BREAKFAST	Calories	Totals
Tomato juice (½ cup)	20	
Shredded Wheat (1 cup) + ½ cup skim milk + ½ banana	265	
Coffee	10	295 Cal
SNACK		
Small bunch of grapes	65	65 Cal
LUNCH		
Roast beef (2 oz) with lettuce sandwich	300	
Hot or iced tea	10	310 Cal
SNACK		
Coffee or tea	10	10 Cal
DINNER		
Pasta Rapini (Day 34 Recipe - page 141)	290	
Small salad with 1 Tbsp dressing	75	
Italian or French bread (1 slice)	80	
Water	0	445 Cal
SNACK		
Fiber One Chocolate Fudge Brownie	90	90 Cal
		1215 Cal

Day 35 – 1200 Calorie Meal Plan

BREAKFAST	Calories	Totals
Cantaloupe (½ medium)	**50**	
Oatmeal (½ cup dry) + ½ cup skim milk + 15 raisins	**220**	
Coffee	**10**	**280 Cal**
SNACK		
Coffee or tea	**10**	**10 Cal**
LUNCH		
Grilled cheese sandwich (2 slices 2% cheese)	**240**	
Diet soda or water	**0**	**240 Cal**
SNACK		
Fresh fruit in season (apple, plum, etc)	**70**	**70 Cal**
DINNER		
Eat Out – Chicken dinner (Day 35 Recipe page 142)	**480**	
Glass of wine (4 oz)	**100**	**580 Cal**
SNACK		
Coffee or tea	**10**	**10 Cal**
		1190 Cal

Day 36 – 1200 Calorie Meal Plan

BREAKFAST	Calories	Totals
Cantaloupe (½ medium)	50	
Wheaties (¾ cup) + ½ cup skim milk + ½ banana	190	
Coffee	10	250 Cal
SNACK		
Coffee or tea	10	10 Cal
LUNCH		
Soup #3 (Appendix C - page 205)	120	
Turkey (1 oz) on 1 slice of rye bread (½ sandwich)	120	
Hot or ice tea	10	250 Cal
SNACK		
Fresh fruit in season (apple, pear, etc)	70	70 Cal
DINNER		
Grilled Tilapia (Day 36 Recipe - page 143)	300	
Asparagus spear (6)	25	
Wild rice (½ cup – after cooking)	100	
Small salad with 1 Tbsp dressing	75	
Glass of wine	100	600 Cal
SNACK		
Coffee or tea	10	10 Cal
		1190 Cal

Day 37 – 1200 Calorie Meal Plan

BREAKFAST	Calories	Totals
Orange juice (½ cup)	50	
Soft-boiled egg	80	
Whole grain toast (1 slice)	70	
Coffee	10	210 Cal
SNACK		
Greek Yogurt (6 oz, nonfat, any flavor)	90	90 Cal
LUNCH		
Salad (3 oz canned tuna, 1 tsp Evoo, onions, celery)	175	
Lettuce & tomato wedges	20	
Italian or French bread (1 slice)	80	
Water	0	275 Cal
SNACK		
Fresh fruit in season (apple, plum, etc)	70	70 Cal
DINNER		
Crab Cakes (Day 37 Recipe - page 144)	320	
Large salad with 2 Tbsp dressing	150	
Glass of wine	100	570 Cal
SNACK		
Coffee or tea	10	10 Cal
		1215 Cal

Day 38 – 1200 Calorie Meal Plan

BREAKFAST	Calories	Totals
Cantaloupe (½ medium)	50	
Fried egg	80	
Toasted raisin bread (1 slice)	75	
Coffee	10	215 Cal
SNACK		
Coffee or tea	10	10 Cal
LUNCH		
Peanut butter (2 Tbsp) on 2 slices bread	340	
Skim milk (4 oz)	45	385 Cal
SNACK		
Coffee or tea	10	10 Cal
DINNER		
Pan-broiled lamb chop (Day 38 Recipe - page 145)	320	
Large salad with 2 Tbsp dressing	150	
Glass of wine	100	570 Cal
SNACK		
Coffee or tea	10	10 Cal
		1200 Cal

Day 39 – 1200 Calorie Meal Plan

BREAKFAST	Calories	Totals
Fresh sliced orange	75	
Cheerios (1 cup) + ½ cup skim milk + about 15 raisins	190	
Coffee	10	275 Cal
SNACK		
Coffee or tea	10	10 Cal
LUNCH		
Cottage cheese (1 cup low fat)	180	
Small salad with 1 Tbsp dressing	75	
Italian or French bread	80	
Hot or iced tea	10	345 Cal
SNACK		
Fresh fruit in season (apple, plum, etc)	70	70 Cal
DINNER		
Chicken with veggies (Day 39 Recipe - page 146)	365	
Glass of wine	100	
Coffee or tea	10	475 Cal
SNACK		
Coffee or tea	10	10 Cal
		1185 Cal

Day 40 – 1200 Calorie Meal Plan

BREAKFAST	Calories	Totals
Grapefruit (½)	75	
Scrambled egg	80	
Toasted raisin bread (1 slice)	75	
Coffee	10	240 Cal
SNACK		
Greek Yogurt (6 oz, nonfat, any flavor)	90	90 Cal
LUNCH		
Soup #8 (Appendix C - page 205)	170	
Italian or French bread (1 slice)	80	
Hot or iced tea	10	260 Cal
SNACK		
Coffee or tea	10	10 Cal
DINNER		
Eat Out – Fish dinner (Day 40 Recipe - page 147)	495	
Glass of wine (4 oz)	100	595 Cal
SNACK		
Coffee or tea	10	10 Cal
		1205 Cal

Day 41 – 1200 Calorie Meal Plan

BREAKFAST	Calories	Totals
Orange juice (½ cup)	50	
Shredded Wheat (1 cup) + ½ cup skim milk + ½	260	
Coffee	10	320 Cal
SNACK		
Coffee or tea	10	10 Cal
LUNCH		
Turkey frank (2 oz) with mustard & relish	150	
Hot dog bun	130	
Diet soda or water	0	280 Cal
SNACK		
Coffee or tea	10	10 Cal
DINNER		
Tina's Frittata (Day 41 Recipe - page 148)	320	
Large salad with 2 Tbsp dressing	150	
Italian or French bread (1 slice)	80	
Water	0	550 Cal
SNACK		
Coffee or tea	10	10 Cal
		1180 Cal

Day 42 – 1200 Calorie Meal Plan

BREAKFAST	Calories	Totals
Cantaloupe (½ medium)	50	
Wheaties (¾ cup) + ½ cup skim milk + ½ banana	190	
Coffee	10	250 Cal
SNACK		
Coffee or tea	10	10 Cal
LUNCH		
Grilled Swiss cheese sandwich (2 oz low-fat cheese)	310	
Pickle spear	0	
Hot or iced tea	10	320 Cal
SNACK		
Coffee or tea	10	10 Cal
DINNER		
Frozen chicken dinner (Day 28 Recipe - page 135)	300	
Large salad with 2 Tbsp dressing	150	
Water with lemon wedge	10	460 Cal
SNACK		
Blueberry Muffin (Day 42 Recipe - page 149)	145	
Coffee or tea	10	155 Cal
		1205 Cal

Day 43 – 1200 Calorie Meal Plan

BREAKFAST	Calories	Totals
Fresh or frozen strawberries (½ cup)	25	
Fried egg	80	
Toasted raisin bread (1 slice)	75	
Coffee	10	190 Cal
SNACK		
Greek Yogurt (6 oz, nonfat, any flavor)	90	90 Cal
LUNCH		
Salad (3 oz canned tuna, 1 tsp Evoo, onions, celery)	175	
Lettuce & tomato wedges	20	
Rye bread (1 slice)	70	
Coffee or tea	10	275 Cal
SNACK		
Fresh fruit in season (apple, plum, etc)	70	70 Cal
DINNER		
Beef Kebob with veggies (Day 43 Recipe - page 150)	390	
Italian or French bread (1 slice)	80	
Glass of wine	100	570 Cal
SNACK		
Coffee or tea	10	10 Cal
		1205 Cal

Day 44 – 1200 Calorie Meal Plan

BREAKFAST	Calories	Totals
Orange juice (½ cup)	50	
Kashi GoLean (1 cup) + ½ cup skim milk + ½ banana	235	
Coffee	10	295 Cal
SNACK		
Fresh fruit in season (apple, plum, etc)	70	70 Cal
LUNCH		
Soup #1 (Appendix C - page 205)	110	
Italian or French bread (1 slice)	80	
Hot or iced tea	10	200 Cal
SNACK		
Carrot sticks + ¼ cup low-fat cottage cheese & chives	60	60 Cal
DINNER		
Baked Haddock (Day 44 Recipe - page 151)	420	
Large salad with 2 Tbsp dressing	150	
Glass of wine	100	475 Cal
SNACK		
Handful unsalted mixed nuts	100	100 Cal
		1200 Cal

Day 45 – 1200 Calorie Meal Plan

BREAKFAST	Calories	Totals
Cantaloupe (½ medium)	50	
Scrambled egg	80	
Toasted whole-grain bread (1 slice)	70	
Coffee	10	210 Cal
SNACK		
Greek Yogurt (6 oz nonfat, any flavor)	90	90 Cal
LUNCH		
Soup #9 (Appendix C - page 205)	180	
Lettuce & tomato sandwich (1 Tbsp light mayo)	170	
Water	0	350 Cal
SNACK		
Coffee or tea	10	10 Cal
DINNER		
Chicken Cacciatore (Day 45 Recipe - page 152)	310	
Italian or French bread (1 slice)	80	
Water	0	390 Cal
SNACK		
Blueberry muffin	145	
Coffee or tea	10	155 Cal
		1205 Cal

Day 46 – 1200 Calorie Meal Plan

BREAKFAST	Calories	Totals
Grapefruit (½)	75	
Cheerios (1 cup) + ½ cup skim milk + about 15	190	
Coffee	10	275 Cal
SNACK		
Coffee or tea	10	10 Cal
LUNCH		
Subway 6" Sandwich (Ham, Cheese + veggies)*	260	
Diet soda or water	0	260 Cal
SNACK		
Coffee or tea	10	10 Cal
DINNER		
Poached Cod (Day 46 Recipe - page 153)	275	
Grilled potatoes	100	
Grilled cherry tomatoes	45	
Spinach (½ cup) steamed with garlic & drizzled	50	
Water with lemon wedge	10	480 Cal
SNACK		
Blueberry muffin	145	
Coffee or tea	10	155 Cal
		1190 Cal

Day 47 – 1200 Calorie Meal Plan

BREAKFAST	Calories	Totals
Grapefruit (½)	75	
Fried egg	80	
Whole-grain toast (1 slice)	70	
Coffee	10	235 Cal
SNACK		
Fresh fruit in season (apple, plum, etc)	70	70 Cal
LUNCH		
Salad (3 oz canned tuna, 1 tsp Evoo, onions, celery)	175	
Lettuce & tomato wedges	20	
Rye bread (1 slice)	70	
Coffee or tea	10	275 Cal
SNACK		
Coffee or tea	10	10 Cal
DINNER		
Black-eyed peas & Rice (Day 47 Recipe - page 154)	280	
Small salad with 1 Tbsp dressing	75	
Glass of wine	100	455 Cal
SNACK		
Blueberry muffin	145	
Coffee or tea	10	155 Cal
		1200 Cal

Day 48 – 1200 Calorie Meal Plan

BREAKFAST	Calories	Totals
Cantaloupe (½ medium)	50	
Oatena cereal mix (Day 14 Recipe - page 121)	310	
Coffee	10	370 Cal
SNACK		
Coffee or tea	10	10 Cal
LUNCH		
Subway 6" Sandwich (Ham, Cheese + veggies)	260	
Diet soda or water	0	260 Cal
SNACK		
Coffee or tea	10	10 Cal
DINNER		
Pasta Salad (Day 48 Recipe - page 155)	370	
Italian or French bread (1 slice)	80	
Glass of wine (4 oz)	100	550 Cal
SNACK		
Coffee or tea	10	10 Cal
		1210 Cal

Day 49 – 1200 Calorie Meal Plan

BREAKFAST	Calories	Totals
Cantaloupe (½ medium)	50	
Oatmeal (½ cup dry) + ½ cup skim milk + about 15	220	
Coffee	10	280 Cal
SNACK		
Greek Yogurt (6 oz nonfat, any flavor)	90	90 Cal
LUNCH		
Turkey breast (2 oz) on 2 slices whole-grain bread	245	
Lettuce, tomato and 1 Tbsp light mayo	35	
Water with lemon wedge	10	290 Cal
SNACK		
Coffee or tea	10	10 Cal
DINNER		
Frozen meat dinner (Day 49 Recipe - page 156)	300	
Small salad with 1 Tbsp dressing	75	
Water with lemon wedge	10	385 Cal
SNACK		
Blueberry muffin	145	
Coffee or tea	10	155 Cal
		1210 Cal

Day 50 – 1200 Calorie Meal Plan

BREAKFAST	Calories	Totals
Fresh or frozen strawberries (1 cup)	25	
French toasted English Muffin (Day 2 Recipe p 109)	270	
Light syrup (1 Tbsp)	30	
Coffee	10	335 Cal
SNACK		
Fresh fruit in season (apple, peach, etc)	70	
Coffee or tea	10	80 Cal
LUNCH		
Soup (Appendix C - page 205)	100	
BLT sandwich (2 slices turkey bacon, 1 Tbsp light mayo)	245	
Hot or iced tea	10	355 Cal
SNACK		
Coffee or tea	10	10 Cal
DINNER		
Pan-fried Sole (Day 50 Recipe - page 157)	325	
Small salad with 1 Tbsp dressing	75	
Water	0	400 Cal
SNACK		
Coffee or tea	10	10 Cal
		1190 Cal

Day 51 – 1200 Calorie Meal Plan

BREAKFAST	Calories	Totals
Cantaloupe (½ medium)	50	
Wheaties (¾ cup) + ½ cup skim milk + ½ banana	190	
Coffee	10	250 Cal
SNACK		
Coffee or tea	10	10 Cal
LUNCH		
Ham (2 oz) with mustard on 2 slices rye bread	290	
Hot or iced tea	10	300 Cal
SNACK		
Handful unsalted mixed nuts	100	
Coffee or tea	10	110 Cal
DINNER		
Beans and Greens Salad (Day 51 Recipe - page 158)	260	
Whole-grain bread (1 slice)	70	
Baked potato (medium)	100	
Water with lemon wedge	10	510 Cal
SNACK		
Coffee or tea	10	10 Cal
		1190 Cal

Day 52 – 1200 Calorie Meal Plan

BREAKFAST	Calories	Totals
Fresh orange sliced	75	
Soft-boiled egg	80	
Whole-grain toast (2 slices)	140	
Coffee	10	305 Cal
SNACK		
Greek Yogurt (6 oz nonfat, any flavor)	90	90 Cal
LUNCH		
Salad – 3 oz canned salmon, 1 tsp Evoo, onions & celery	200	
Lettuce & tomato wedges	20	
Italian or French bread (1 slice)	70	
Water	0	290 Cal
SNACK		
Fresh fruit in season (apple, plum, etc)	70	
DINNER		
Chicken Piccata (Day 52 Recipe - page 159)	270	
Brown rice (½ cup – after cooking)	100	
Small salad with 1 Tbsp dressing	75	
Water	0	445 Cal
SNACK		
Coffee or tea	10	10 Cal
		1210 Cal

Day 53 – 1200 Calorie Meal Plan

BREAKFAST	Calories	Totals
Grapefruit (½)	75	
Cheerios (1 cup) + ½ cup skim milk + about 15 raisins	190	
Coffee	10	275 Cal
SNACK		
Fresh fruit in season (peach, plum, etc)	70	
Coffee or tea	10	80 Cal
LUNCH		
Cottage cheese (1 cup low fat)	180	
Small salad with 1 Tbsp dressing	75	
Hot or iced tea	10	265 Cal
SNACK		
Coffee or tea	10	10 Cal
DINNER		
Pasta Primavera (Day 53 Recipe - page 160)	350	
Italian or French bread (1 slice)	80	
Glass of wine (4 oz)	100	530 Cal
SNACK		
Coffee or tea	10	10 Cal
		1170 Cal

Day 54 – 1200 Calorie Meal Plan

BREAKFAST	Calories	Totals
Cantaloupe (½ medium)	50	
Fried egg	80	
Toasted whole-grain bread (1 slice)	70	
Coffee	10	210 Cal
SNACK		
Greek Yogurt (6 oz nonfat, any flavor)	90	90 Cal
LUNCH		
Soup #10 (Appendix C - page 205)	200	
Italian or French bread (1 slice)	80	
Lettuce & tomato slices	20	
Water	0	300 Cal
SNACK		
Coffee or tea	10	10 Cal
DINNER		
Grilled scallops (Day 54 Recipe - page 161)	210	
Grilled polenta (Day 54 Recipe)	125	
Mushroom-steamed green beans - (Day 54 Recipe)	45	
Grilled asparagus (Day 54 Recipe)	10	
Large salad with 2 Tbsp dressing	150	
Water	0	540 Cal
SNACK		
Fresh fruit in season (apple, peach, etc)	70	70 Cal
		1220 Cal

Day 55 – 1200 Calorie Meal Plan

BREAKFAST	Calories	Totals
Cantaloupe (½ medium)	50	
Oatmeal (½ cup dry) + ½ cup skim milk + about 15 raisins	220	
Coffee	10	280 Cal
SNACK		
Fresh fruit in season (apple, peach, etc)	70	70 Cal
LUNCH		
Two servings (1 cup) of left over Day 51 salad	270	
Small whole-grain roll	80	
Lettuce & tomato slices	20	
Hot or iced tea	10	380 Cal
SNACK		
Coffee or tea	10	10 Cal
DINNER		
Hearty Vegetable Soup (Day 55 Recipe - page 162)	360	
Italian or French bread (1 slice)	80	
Water	0	440 Cal
SNACK		
Coffee or tea	10	10 Cal
		1190 Cal

Day 56 – 1200 Calorie Meal Plan

BREAKFAST	Calories	Totals
Tomato juice (½ cup)	20	
Shredded Wheat (1 cup) + ½ cup skim milk + ½ banana	260	
Coffee	10	290 Cal
SNACK		
Fresh fruit in season (pear, plum, etc)	70	70 Cal
LUNCH		
Roast beef (2 oz) sandwich on whole-grain bread	305	
Lettuce	0	
Diet soda or water	0	305 Cal
SNACK		
Coffee or tea	10	10 Cal
DINNER		
Frozen chicken dinner (Day 56 Recipe - page 163)	300	
Small salad with 1 Tbsp dressing	75	
Whole-grain bread (1 slice)	70	
Water	0	445 Cal
SNACK		
Graham crackers (2 squares)	60	
Coffee or tea	10	70 Cal
		1190 Cal

Day 57 – 1200 Calorie Meal Plan

BREAKFAST	Calories	Totals
Cantaloupe (½ medium)	50	
Oatena cereal mix (Day 14 Recipe - page 121)	310	
Coffee	10	370 Cal
SNACK		
Coffee or tea	10	10 Cal
LUNCH		
Salad (3 oz canned tuna, 1 tsp Evoo, onions, celery)	175	
Lettuce & tomato wedges	20	
Italian or French bread (1 slice)	75	
Water	0	270 Cal
SNACK		
Coffee or tea	10	10 Cal
DINNER		
Salmon with Mango Salsa (Day 57 Recipe - p 164)	460	
Small salad with 1 Tbsp dressing	75	
Water with lemon wedge	10	545 Cal
SNACK		
Coffee or tea	10	10 Cal
		1215 Cal

Day 58 – 1200 Calorie Meal Plan

BREAKFAST	Calories	Totals
Tomato juice (½ cup)	20	
Kashi GoLean (1 cup) + ½ cup skim milk + ½ banana	235	
Coffee	10	265 Cal
SNACK		
Coffee or tea	10	10 Cal
LUNCH		
Soup #2 (Appendix C - page 205)	120	
Italian or French bread (1 slice)	80	
Hot or iced tea	10	200 Cal
SNACK		
Coffee or tea	10	10 Cal
DINNER		
Grilled pork chop with orange (Day 58 Recipe p 165)	470	
Wild rice (¼ cup – after cooking)	50	
Asparagus (7 spear cooked & drained)	20	
Water with lemon wedge	10	550 Cal
SNACK		
Blueberry muffin	145	
Coffee or tea	10	155 Cal
		1190 Cal

Day 59 – 1200 Calorie Meal Plan

BREAKFAST	Calories	Totals
Grapefruit (½)	75	
Scrambled egg	80	
Whole-grain toast (1 slice)	70	
Coffee	10	235 Cal
SNACK		
Fresh fruit in season (peach, plum, etc)	70	70 Cal
LUNCH		
Soup #5 (Appendix C - page 205)	140	
Tomato slices + ¼ cup chopped basil + 1 tsp Evoo	50	
Italian or French bread (1 slice)	80	
Hot or ice tea	10	280 Cal
SNACK		
Coffee or tea	10	10 Cal
DINNER		
Eat Out – Fish dinner (Day 59 Recipe - page 166)	495	
Glass of wine (4 oz)	100	595 Cal
SNACK		
Coffee or tea	10	10 Cal
		1200 Cal

Day 60 – 1200 Calorie Meal Plan

BREAKFAST	Calories	Totals
Grapefruit (½)	75	
Cheerios (1 cup) + ½ cup skim milk + about 15 raisins	190	
Coffee	10	275 Cal
SNACK		
Coffee or tea	10	10 Cal
LUNCH		
Subway 6" Sandwich (Ham, Cheese + veggies)*	260	
Water or diet soda	0	260 Cal
SNACK		
Coffee or tea	10	10 Cal
DINNER		
Chicken Stew (Day 60 Recipe - page 167)	360	
Brown rice (½ cup – after cooking)	100	
Italian or French bread (1 slice)	80	
Glass of wine (4 oz)	100	640 Cal
SNACK		
Coffee or tea	10	10 Cal
		1205 Cal

Day 61 – 1200 Calorie Meal Plan

BREAKFAST	Calories	Totals
Orange juice (½ cup)	50	
Wheaties (¾ cup) + ½ cup skim milk + ½ banana	190	
Coffee	10	250 Cal
SNACK		
Fresh fruit in season (apple, plum, etc)	70	70 Cal
LUNCH		
Soup (Appendix C - page 205)	110	
Turkey breast (1 oz) 1 slice rye bread (½ sandwich)	105	
Lettuce & tomato slices	20	
Water	0	235 Cal
SNACK		
Coffee or tea	10	10 Cal
DINNER		
Shrimp over Spaghetti (Day 61 Recipe - page 168)	450	
Small salad with 1 Tbsp dressing	75	
Glass of wine (4 oz)	100	625 Cal
SNACK		
Coffee or tea	10	10 Cal
		1200 Cal

Day 62 – 1200 Calorie Meal Plan

BREAKFAST	Calories	Totals
Tomato juice (½ cup)	20	
French toasted English Muffin (Day 2 Recipe p 109)	270	
Light syrup (1 Tbsp)	30	
Coffee	10	330 Cal
SNACK		
Fresh fruit in season (apple, pear, etc)	70	70 Cal
LUNCH		
Salad (3 oz canned tuna, 1 tsp Evoo, onions, celery)	175	
Lettuce & tomato wedges	20	
Italian or French bread (1 slice)	80	
Water	0	275 Cal
SNACK		
Coffee or tea	10	10 Cal
DINNER		
Beef Burgundy (Day 62 Recipe - page 169)	350	
Small salad with 1 Tbsp dressing	75	
Glass of wine (4 oz)	100	525 Cal
SNACK		
Coffee or tea	10	10 Cal
		1220 Cal

Day 63 – 1200 Calorie Meal Plan

BREAKFAST	Calories	Totals
Grapefruit (½)	75	
Scrambled egg	80	
Whole grain toast (1 slice)	70	
Coffee	10	235 Cal
SNACK		
Yogurt (6 oz nonfat, any flavor)	90	90 Cal
LUNCH		
Ham (2 oz) with mustard on 2 slices rye bread	290	
Diet soda or water	0	290 Cal
SNACK		
Coffee or tea	10	10 Cal
DINNER		
Chicken cutlet (Day 63 Recipe - page 170)	450	
One small baked potato	50	
Small salad with 1 Tbsp dressing*	70	
Water	0	570 Cal
* Note Day 63 recipe shows much of salad on dinner plate		
SNACK		
Coffee or tea	10	10 Cal
		1205 Cal

Day 64 – 1200 Calorie Meal Plan

BREAKFAST	Calories	Totals
Grapefruit (½)	75	
Cheerios (1 cup) + ½ cup skim milk + ½ banana	210	
Coffee	10	295 Cal
SNACK		
Fresh fruit in season (apple, pear, etc)	70	70 Cal
LUNCH		
Cottage cheese (1 cup low fat)	180	
Small salad with 1 Tbsp dressing	75	
Water	0	255 Cal
SNACK		
Coffee or tea	10	10 Cal
DINNER		
Turkey Meat Loaf (Day 64 Recipe - page 171)	240	
Brown rice (½ cup – after cooking)	100	
Green beans - steamed	30	
Glass of wine (4 oz)	100	470 Cal
SNACK		
100-Calorie Pack Cookies*	100	
Coffee or tea	10	110 Cal
* Such as, Nabisco Oreo/Chips Ahoy/etc.		1210 Cal

Day 65 – 1200 Calorie Meal Plan

BREAKFAST	Calories	Totals
Cantaloupe (½ medium)	50	
Oatena cereal mix (Day 14 Recipe - page 121)	310	
Coffee	10	370 Cal
SNACK		
Coffee or tea	10	10 Cal
LUNCH		
Soup #1 (Appendix C - page 205)	110	
Italian or French bread (1 slice)	80	
Hot or ice tea	10	230 Cal
SNACK		
Coffee or tea	10	10 Cal
DINNER		
Frozen fish dinner (Day 65 Recipe - page 172)	340	
Small salad with 1 Tbsp dressing	75	
Whole-grain bread (1 slice)	70	
Glass of wine (4 oz)	100	585 Cal
SNACK		
Coffee or tea	10	10 Cal
		1215 Cal

Day 66 – 1200 Calorie Meal Plan

BREAKFAST	Calories	Totals
Tomato juice (½ cup)	20	
Shredded Wheat (1 cup) + ½ cup skim milk + ½ banana	265	
Coffee	10	295 Cal
SNACK		
Fresh fruit in season (peach, plum, etc)	70	70 Cal
LUNCH		
Salad – 3 oz canned salmon, 1 tsp Evoo, onions & celery	200	
Lettuce & tomato wedges	20	
Italian or French bread (1 slice)	80	
Hot or ice tea	10	310 Cal
SNACK		
Coffee or tea	10	10 Cal
DINNER		
Pita Pizza (Day 66 Recipe - page 173)	430	
Small salad with 1 Tbsp dressing	75	
Water	0	505 Cal
SNACK		
Coffee or tea	10	10 Cal
		1200 Cal

Day 67 – 1200 Calorie Meal Plan

BREAKFAST	Calories	Totals
Cantaloupe (½ medium)	50	
Oatmeal (½ cup dry) + ½ cup skim milk	190	
Coffee	10	250 Cal
SNACK		
Coffee or tea	10	10 Cal
LUNCH		
Soup #3 (Appendix C - page 205)	120	
Grilled cheese sandwich (2 slices 2% cheese)	240	
Diet soda or water	0	360 Cal
SNACK		
Coffee or tea	10	10 Cal
DINNER		
Eat Out – Chicken dinner (Day 67 Recipe p 174)	480	
Glass of wine (4 oz)	100	580 Cal
SNACK		
Coffee or tea	10	10 Cal
		1220 Cal

Day 68 – 1200 Calorie Meal Plan

BREAKFAST	Calories	Totals
Cantaloupe (½ medium)	50	
Wheaties (¾ cup) + ½ cup skim milk + ½ banana	190	
Coffee	10	250 Cal
SNACK		
Coffee or tea	10	10 Cal
LUNCH		
Soup #7 (Appendix C - page 205)	160	
Turkey (1 oz) on 1 slice of rye bread (½ sandwich)	120	
Lettuce	0	
Water	0	280 Cal
SNACK		
Coffee or tea	10	10 Cal
DINNER		
Pork Medallions lime sauce (Day 68 Recipe p 175)	450	
Green beans - steamed	25	
Small salad with 1 Tbsp dressing	75	
Glass of wine (4 oz)	100	650 Cal
SNACK		
Coffee or tea	10	10 Cal
		1210 Cal

Day 69 – 1200 Calorie Meal Plan

BREAKFAST	Calories	Totals
Orange juice (½ cup)	50	
Soft-boiled egg	80	
Whole grain toast (1 slice)	70	
Coffee	10	210 Cal
SNACK		
Greek Yogurt (6 oz nonfat, any flavor)	90	90 Cal
LUNCH		
Salad (3 oz canned tuna, 1 tsp Evoo, onions, celery)	175	
Lettuce & tomato wedges + rye bread (1 slice)	90	
Coffee or tea	10	345 Cal
SNACK		
Fresh fruit in season – (apple, peach, etc)	70	70 Cal
DINNER		
Healthy Chicken Salad (Day 69 Recipe - page 176)	330	
Italian or French bread (1 slice)	80	
Water with lemon wedge	10	420 Cal
SNACK		
Graham crackers (2 squares)	60	
Coffee or tea	10	70 Cal
		1205 Cal

Day 70 – 1200 Calorie Meal Plan

BREAKFAST	Calories	Totals
Orange juice (½ cup)	50	
Wild blueberry pancakes (Day 10 Recipe - page 117)	190	
Light syrup (1½ Tbsp)	45	
Coffee	10	295 Cal
SNACK		
Fresh fruit in season (apple, peach, etc)	70	
Coffee or tea	10	80 Cal
LUNCH		
Peanut butter (2 Tbsp) on 2 slices whole-grain bread	340	
Skim milk (6 oz)	70	410 Cal
SNACK		
Coffee or tea	10	10 Cal
DINNER		
Baked Cod (Day 70 Recipe - page 177)	230	
Brown rice (½ cup – after cooking)	100	
Green beans - steamed	25	
Zucchini, tomatoes & onion – steamed	45	
Water	0	400 Cal
SNACK		
Coffee or tea	10	10 Cal
		1205 Cal

Day 71 – 1200 Calorie Meal Plan

BREAKFAST	Calories	Totals
Fresh sliced orange	75	
Cheerios (1 cup) + ½ cup skim milk + about 15 raisins	190	
Coffee	10	275 Cal
SNACK		
Coffee or tea	10	10 Cal
LUNCH		
Cottage cheese (1 cup low fat)	180	
Small salad with 1 Tbsp dressing	75	
Italian or French bread (1 slice)	80	
Hot or iced tea	10	345 Cal
SNACK		
Coffee or tea	10	10 Cal
DINNER		
Chicken Scaloppini (Day 71 Recipe - page 178)	260	
White Rice (½ cup – after cooking)	100	
Snow peas or green beans - steamed	25	
Glass of wine (4 oz)	100	485 Cal
SNACK		
Graham crackers (2 squares)	60	
Coffee or tea	10	70 Cal
		1195 Cal

Day 72 – 1200 Calorie Meal Plan

BREAKFAST	Calories	Totals
Grapefruit (½)	75	
Scrambled egg	80	
Whole-grain toast (1 slice)	70	
Coffee	10	235 Cal
SNACK		
Greek Yogurt (6 oz nonfat, any flavor)	90	90 Cal
LUNCH		
Soup #7 (Appendix C - page 205)	160	
Italian or French bread (1 slice)	80	
Hot or iced tea	10	250 Cal
SNACK		
Coffee or tea	10	10 Cal
DINNER		
Eat Out – Fish dinner (Day 72 Recipe - page 179)	495	
Glass of wine (4 oz)	100	595 Cal
SNACK		
Coffee or tea	10	10 Cal
		1190 Cal

Day 73 – 1200 Calorie Meal Plan

BREAKFAST	Calories	Totals
Orange juice (½ cup)	50	
Shredded Wheat (1 cup)+ ½ cup skim milk + ½ banana	260	
Coffee	10	320 Cal
SNACK		
Coffee or tea	10	10 Cal
LUNCH		
Turkey frank (2 oz) with mustard & relish	150	
Hot-dog bun	130	
Diet soda or water	0	280 Cal
SNACK		
Coffee or tea	10	10 Cal
DINNER		
Pasta Pomodoro (Day 73 Recipe - page 180)	420	
Small salad with 1 Tbsp dressing	75	
Italian or French bread (1 slice)	80	
Water with lemon wedge	10	585 Cal
SNACK		
Coffee or tea	10	10 Cal
		1215 Cal

Day 74 – 1200 Calorie Meal Plan

BREAKFAST	Calories	Totals
Cantaloupe (½ medium)	50	
Wheaties (¾ cup) + ½ cup skim milk + ½ banana	190	
Coffee	10	250 Cal
SNACK		
Fresh fruit in season (peach, plum, etc)	70	70 Cal
LUNCH		
Grilled Swiss cheese sandwich (2 oz low-fat cheese)	320	
Hot or iced tea	10	330 Cal
SNACK		
Coffee or tea	10	10 Cal
DINNER		
Frozen chicken dinner (Day 74 Recipe - page 181)	300	
Small salad with 1 Tbsp dressing	75	
Glass of wine (4 oz)	100	475 Cal
SNACK		
Graham crackers (2 squares)	60	
Coffee or tea	10	70 Cal
		1205 Cal

Day 75 – 1200 Calorie Meal Plan

BREAKFAST	Calories	Totals
Cantaloupe (½ medium)	50	
Oatena cereal mix (Day 14 Recipe - page 121)	310	
Coffee	10	370 Cal
SNACK		
Fresh fruit in season (peach, plum, etc)	70	70 Cal
LUNCH		
Subway 6" Sandwich (Roast Beef, Cheese + veggies)	245	
Diet soda or water	0	245 Cal
SNACK		
Coffee or tea	10	10 Cal
DINNER		
Mediterranean Chicken (Day 75 Recipe - p. 182)	200	
Spaghetti squash (1 cup steamed & drizzled with 1	90	
Green beans (¼ lb – steamed)	25	
Italian or French bread (1 slice)	80	
Glass of wine (4 oz)	100	495 Cal
SNACK		
Coffee or tea	10	10 Cal
		1200 Cal

Day 76 – 1200 Calorie Meal Plan

BREAKFAST	Calories	Totals
Orange juice (½ cup)	50	
Kashi GoLean (1 cup) + ½ cup skim milk	185	
Coffee	10	245 Cal
SNACK		
Fresh fruit in season (apple, peach, etc)	70	70 Cal
LUNCH		
Soup #6 (Appendix C - page 205)	150	
Italian or French bread (1 slice)	80	
Hot or iced tea	10	240 Cal
SNACK		
Coffee or tea	10	10 Cal
DINNER		
Grilled Sea Scallops (Day 76 Recipe - page 183)	200	
Corn on the cob – one ear	100	
Tomato slices drizzled with Evoo	60	
Small salad with 1 Tbsp dressing	75	
Glass of wine (4 oz)	100	535 Cal
SNACK		
Graham crackers (3 squares)	90	
Coffee or tea	10	100 Cal
		1200 Cal

Day 77 – 1200 Calorie Meal Plan

BREAKFAST	Calories	Totals
Cantaloupe (½ medium)	50	
Fried egg	80	
Toasted raisin bread (1 slice)	75	
Coffee	10	215 Cal
SNACK		
Coffee or tea	10	10 Cal
LUNCH		
Soup #7 (Appendix C - page 205)	160	
Lettuce & tomato sandwich (Tbsp light mayo)	180	
Cucumber slices and carrots and celery sticks	15	
Water	0	355 Cal
SNACK		
Fresh fruit in season (apple, peach, etc)	70	70 Cal
DINNER		
Chicken w Peppers & Rice (Day 77 Recipe - p 184)	290	
Small salad with 1 Tbsp dressing	75	
Italian or French bread (1 slice)	80	
Glass of wine (4 oz)	100	545 Cal
SNACK		
Coffee or tea	10	10 Cal
		1205 Cal

Day 78 – 1200 Calorie Meal Plan

BREAKFAST	Calories	Totals
Grapefruit (½)	75	
Cheerios (1 cup) + ½ cup skim milk + about 15 raisins	190	
Coffee	10	275 Cal
SNACK		
Coffee or tea	10	10 Cal
LUNCH		
Soup #9 (Appendix C - page 205)	180	
Small salad with 1 Tbsp dressing	75	
Italian or French bread (1 slice)	80	
Hot or iced tea	10	345 Cal
SNACK		
Coffee or tea	10	10 Cal
DINNER		
Trout with Lemon Capers (Day 78 Recipe - p 185)	340	
Wild rice (½ cup – after cooking)	100	
Green beans (steamed)	30	
Sautéed cherry tomatoes (See page 132)	60	
Water with lemon wedge	10	540 Cal
SNACK		
Coffee or tea	10	10 Cal
		1190 Cal

Day 79 – 1200 Calorie Meal Plan

BREAKFAST	Calories	Totals
Grapefruit (½)	75	
Scrambled egg	80	
Whole-grain toast (1 slice)	70	
Coffee	10	235 Cal
SNACK		
Small bunch of grapes	65	65 Cal
LUNCH		
Subway 6" Sandwich (Ham, Cheese + veggies)	260	
Diet soda or water	0	260 Cal
SNACK		
Coffee or tea	10	10 Cal
DINNER		
Eat Out – Italian food (Day 79 Recipe - page 186)	540	
Glass of wine (4 oz)	100	640 Cal
SNACK		
Coffee or tea	10	10 Cal
		1220 Cal

Day 80 – 1200 Calorie Meal Plan

BREAKFAST	Calories	Totals
Tomato juice (½ cup)	20	
Shredded Wheat (1 cup) + ½ cup milk + ½ banana	260	
Coffee	10	290 Cal
SNACK		
Coffee or tea	10	10 Cal
LUNCH		
Left over Chinese food from Day 79	260	
Hot or iced tea	10	270 Cal
SNACK		
Coffee or tea	10	10 Cal
DINNER		
Vegetable Chili (Day 80 Recipe - page 187)	360	
Brown rice (½ cup – after cooking)	100	
Small salad with 1 Tbsp dressing	75	
Italian or French bread (1 slice)	80	
Water	0	615 Cal
SNACK		
Coffee or tea	10	10 Cal
		1205 Cal

Day 81 – 1200 Calorie Meal Plan

BREAKFAST	Calories	Totals
Cantaloupe (½ medium)	50	
Oatmeal (½ cup dry) + ½ cup skim milk	190	
Coffee	10	250 Cal
SNACK		
Fresh fruit in season (apple, peach, etc)	70	70 Cal
LUNCH		
Turkey breast (2 oz) sandwich	245	
Lettuce, tomato and Tbsp light mayo	35	
Hot or iced tea	10	290 Cal
SNACK		
Coffee or tea	10	10 Cal
DINNER		
Frozen meat dinner (Day 81 Recipe - page 188)	300	
Small salad with 1 Tbsp dressing	75	
Italian or French bread (1 slice)	80	
Glass of wine (4 oz)	100	555 Cal
SNACK		
Coffee or tea	10	10 Cal
		1185 Cal

Day 82 – 1200 Calorie Meal Plan

BREAKFAST	Calories	Totals
Fresh or frozen strawberries (1 cup)	25	
French toasted English Muffin (Day 2 Recipe p 109)	270	
Light syrup (1 Tbsp)	30	
Coffee	10	335 Cal
SNACK		
Coffee or tea	10	10 Cal
LUNCH		
Soup #3 (Appendix C - page 205)	120	
BLT sandwich (2 slices turkey bacon, 1 Tbsp light mayo)	245	
Hot or iced tea	10	375 Cal
SNACK		
Coffee or tea	10	10 Cal
DINNER		
Chicken Salad (Day 82 Recipe - page 189)	440	
Hot or iced tea	10	450 Cal
SNACK		
Coffee or tea	10	10 Cal
		1190 Cal

Day 83 – 1200 Calorie Meal Plan

BREAKFAST	Calories	Totals
Cantaloupe (½ medium)	50	
Wheaties (¾ cup) + ½ cup skim milk + ½ banana	190	
Coffee	10	250 Cal
SNACK		
Coffee or tea	10	10 Cal
LUNCH		
Ham (2 oz) with mustard on 2 slices rye bread	300	
Hot or iced tea	10	310 Cal
SNACK		
Coffee or tea	10	10 Cal
DINNER		
Hearty Lentil Soup (Day 83 Recipe - page 190)	260	
Small salad with 1 Tbsp dressing	75	
Italian or French bread (1 slice)	80	
Glass of wine (4 oz)	100	515 Cal
SNACK		
100-Calorie Pack Cookies*	100	
Coffee or tea	10	110 Cal
* Such as, Nabisco Oreo/Chips Ahoy/etc.		1205 Cal

Day 84 – 1200 Calorie Meal Plan

BREAKFAST	Calories	Totals
Fresh orange sliced	75	
Soft-boiled egg	80	
Whole-grain toast (1 slice)	70	
Coffee	10	235 Cal
SNACK		
Greek Yogurt (6 oz nonfat, any flavor)	90	90 Cal
LUNCH		
Salad – 3 oz canned salmon, 1 tsp Evoo, onions & celery	200	
Lettuce & tomato wedges	20	
Rye bread (1 slice)	70	
Coffee or tea	10	300 Cal
SNACK		
Coffee or tea	10	10 Cal
DINNER		
Turkey Burger (Day 84 Recipe - page 191)	360	
Green beans or asparagus - steamed	25	
Large tossed salad with 1½ Tbsp low-cal dressing	70	
Water	0	455 Cal
SNACK		
Handful unsalted mixed nuts	100	
Coffee or tea	10	110 Cal
		1200 Cal

Day 85 – 1200 Calorie Meal Plan

BREAKFAST	Calories	Totals
Grapefruit (½)	75	
Cheerios (1 cup) + ½ cup skim milk	160	
Coffee	10	245 Cal
SNACK		
Fresh fruit in season (apple, plum, etc)	70	
Coffee or tea	10	80 Cal
LUNCH		
Cottage cheese (1 cup low fat)	180	
Small salad with 1 Tbsp dressing	75	
Italian or French bread (1 slice)	80	
Water	0	335 Cal
SNACK		
Coffee or tea	10	10 Cal
DINNER		
Meat Loaf (Day 85 Recipe - page 192)	290	
One-half acorn squash (baked with ½ tsp maple syrup)	90	
Spinach (½ cup steamed & drizzled with 1 tsp Evoo)	70	
Whole-grain bread (1 slice)	70	
Water	0	520 Cal
SNACK		
Coffee or tea	10	10 Cal
		1200 Cal

Day 86 – 1200 Calorie Meal Plan

BREAKFAST	Calories	Totals
Cantaloupe (½ medium)	50	
Fried egg	80	
Toasted whole-grain bread (1 slice)	70	
Coffee	10	210 Cal
SNACK		
Yogurt (6 oz nonfat, any flavor)	90	90 Cal
LUNCH		
Soup #10 (Appendix C - page 205)	200	
Italian or French bread (1 slice)	80	
Lettuce & tomato slices	20	
Water	0	300 Cal
SNACK		
Coffee or tea	10	10 Cal
DINNER		
Tuna & Bean Salad (Day 86 Recipe - page 193)	355	
Italian or French bread (1 slice)	80	
Water	0	435 Cal
SNACK		
Blueberry muffin	145	
Coffee or tea	10	155 Cal
		1200 Cal

Day 87 – 1200 Calorie Meal Plan

BREAKFAST	Calories	Totals
Tomato juice (½ cup)	20	
Oatena cereal mix (Day 14 Recipe - page 121)	310	
Coffee	10	340 Cal
SNACK		
Fresh fruit in season (peach, plum, etc)	70	70 Cal
LUNCH		
Leftover meat loaf (½ of Day 85 serving)	145	
Italian or French bread (1 slice)	80	
Lettuce & tomato slices	20	
Water	0	245 Cal
SNACK		
Coffee or tea	10	10 Cal
DINNER		
Pasta Primavera (Day 87 Recipe - page 194)	460	
Small salad with 1 Tbsp dressing	75	
Water	0	535 Cal
SNACK		
Coffee or tea	10	10 Cal
		1210 Cal

Day 88 – 1200 Calorie Meal Plan

BREAKFAST	Calories	Totals
Tomato juice (½ cup)	20	
Shredded Wheat (1 cup) + ½ cup skim milk + ½ banana	260	
Coffee	10	290 Cal
SNACK		
Fresh fruit in season (peach, plum, etc)	70	
Coffee or tea	10	80 Cal
LUNCH		
Subway 6" Sandwich (Ham, Cheese + veggies)	260	
Diet soda or water	0	260 Cal
SNACK		
Handful unsalted mixed nuts	100	
Coffee or tea	10	110 Cal
DINNER		
Frozen chicken dinner (Day 88 Recipe - page 195)	300	
Small salad with 1 Tbsp dressing	75	
Italian or French bread (1 slice)	80	
Water with lemon wedge	10	465 Cal
SNACK		
Coffee or tea	10	10 Cal
		1215 Cal

Day 89 – 1200 Calorie Meal Plan

BREAKFAST	Calories	Totals
Orange juice (½ cup)	50	
Wild blueberry pancakes (Day 10 Recipe - p. 117)	190	
Light syrup (1½ Tbsp)	45	
Coffee	10	295 Cal
SNACK		
Yogurt (6 oz, nonfat, any flavor)	90	90 Cal
LUNCH		
Salad (3 oz canned tuna, 1 tsp Evoo, onions, celery)	175	
Lettuce & tomato wedges	20	
Rye bread (1 slice)	70	
Water	0	265 Cal
SNACK		
Fresh fruit in season (apple, pear, etc)	70	70 Cal
DINNER		
Fish stew (Day 89 Recipe - page 196)	300	
Small salad with 1 Tbsp dressing	75	
Italian or French bread (1 slice)	80	
Water with lemon wedge	10	465 Cal
SNACK		
Coffee or tea	10	10 Cal
		1195 Cal

Day 90 – 1200 Calorie Meal Plan

BREAKFAST	Calories	Totals
Fresh orange sliced	75	
Kashi GoLean (1 cup) + ½ cup skim milk	185	
Coffee	10	270 Cal
SNACK		
Coffee or tea	10	10 Cal
LUNCH		
Soup #5 (Appendix C - page 205)	140	
Whole-grain bread (1 slice)	70	
Hot or iced tea	10	220 Cal
SNACK		
Coffee or tea	10	10 Cal
DINNER		
Veal w Mushrooms & Tomato (Day 90 Recipe)	520	
Italian or French bread (1 slice)	80	
Glass of wine (4 oz)	100	700 Cal
SNACK		
Coffee or tea	10	10 Cal
		1220 Cal

Recipes and Diet Tips

Day 1- Recipe

<u>Chicken with Peppers & Onions</u>

4 boneless and skinless chicken breasts (about 5 oz each)
Coat the chicken breasts in a bottled barbeque sauce. Prepare medium-hot
fire on well-oiled grill. Place breasts on grill, turning them every 4
minutes, for 10 to 12 minutes, or until done. (To check if breasts are done,
the meat should be moist and white with no sign of pink when you cut into
the breast.) Salt and pepper to taste.
2 medium red peppers, sliced
1 medium onion, sliced
Place peppers and onions in pan with 2 tablespoons fat-free chicken stock.
Sauté until stock is reduced. Spray pan lightly with non-stick cooking oil
and cook another 2 minutes. Salt and pepper to taste.
<u>Serves 4</u>. About 250 Calories per serving (for chicken only).

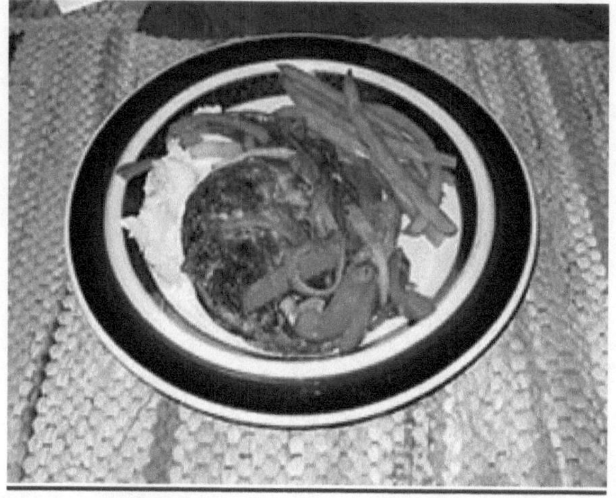

<u>Diet Tip of the Day:</u> Weight Loss – take it one step, one meal, one
workout, one day at a time. Just think of where you'll be in 90 days!

Day 2 Recipe

<u>French-Toasted English Muffin</u>

6 whole wheat English muffins (light)

4 eggs

2 cups skim milk

2 teaspoons (tsp) vanilla

Dash of cinnamon

In a medium bowl, beat together eggs and skim milk. Add vanilla and cinnamon. Separate English muffins into halves and saturate slices in egg mixture. In a non-stick skillet coated with cooking spray, cook muffins until both sides are golden brown. Dust lightly with confectionary sugar. Serve hot or keep in an oven or warmer at 200 ºF until ready to plate. **Serves 4**. Three English muffin slices (1½ muffins) per serving. Serving is 270 Calories.

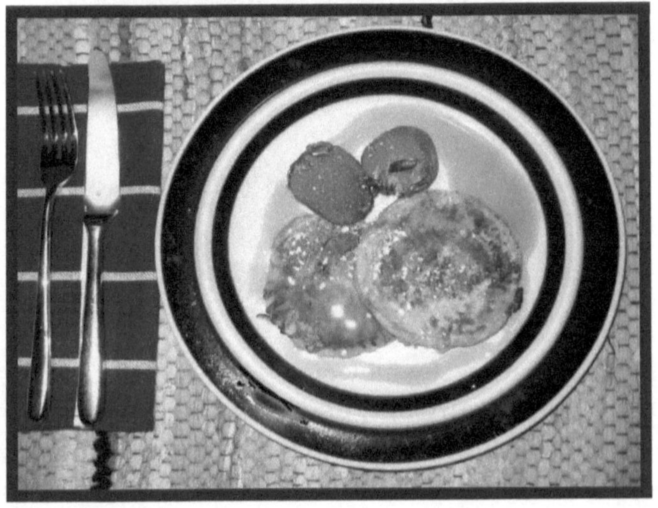

Diet Tip of the Day: "Eat Slowly" This is especially vital when you are trying to lose weight. If you are someone who eats fast, who finishes before everyone else at the table, you are not giving yourself a chance to feel full. While everyone else is still eating, you either sit there and pick, or you have seconds, taking in extra calories you could avoid if you would just slow down.

Day 3 Recipe

<u>Baked Herb-Crusted Cod</u>

 4 cod fish fillets (4 to 5 ounces each)
 2 tablespoons flour
 2 tablespoons cornmeal
 2 tablespoons minced fresh herbs
 2 teaspoons lemon juice

Sprinkle cod with lemon juice. Mix flour, cornmeal and herbs and dust
the cod with the cornmeal-herb mixture. Bake in oven at 375 °F for 10
minutes. Add salt and black pepper to taste.
<u>Serves 4</u>. One serving is about 230 Calories (for cod only).

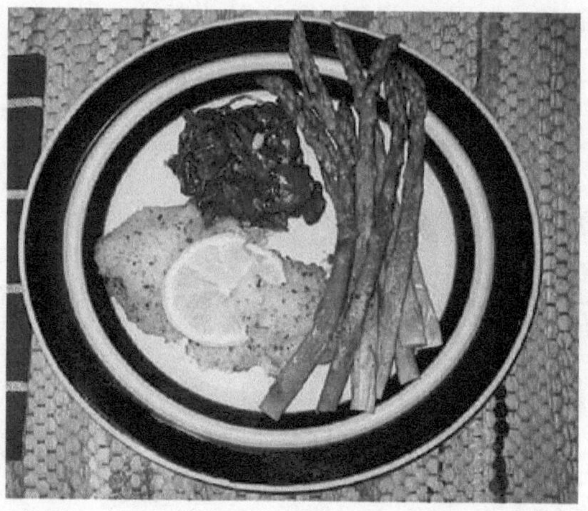

<u>Diet Tip of the Day:</u>. Successful weight loss and subsequent weight
maintenance **requires knowledge, desire and discipline**. Avoid the latest
fad diets. Instead, take the time to develop a true understanding of weight
control and then change your eating and activity habits accordingly.

Day 4 Recipe

Pasta and Veggies

- ¾ pound penne pasta
- 2 cups broccoli florets
- 1 red bell pepper, sliced
- 1 carrot, cut to 1-inch sticks
- ½ cup frozen green peas & ½ cup frozen sweet corn
- 1 small onion, chopped
- 1 tablespoon minced garlic
- 3 tablespoons olive oil
- 1 teaspoon fresh basil, chopped

Cook penne pasta per package directions. Drain and place pasta in a bowl. Pre-cook the carrot and broccoli florets.

In a large heavy skillet, heat the olive oil and sauté onion and garlic until lightly golden. Add vegetables and sauté until the peppers are soft. Combine sautéed vegetables in the bowl with the pasta. Toss well. Garnish with chopped basil, season to taste, and top with freshly grated Parmesan cheese.

Serves 4. 460 Calories per serving

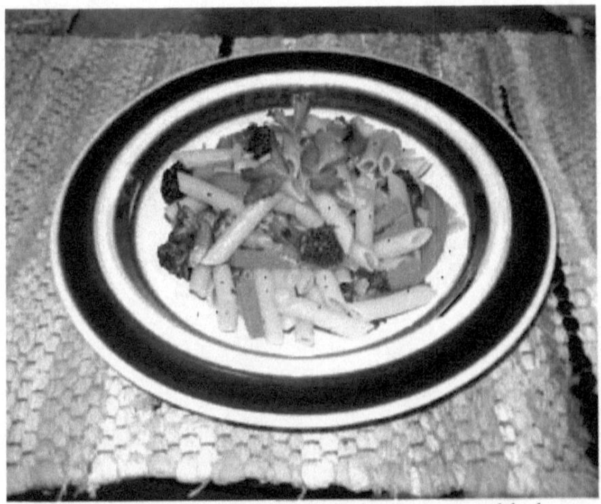

Photo taken before grated cheese was added.

Diet Tip of the Day: When possible, **select fresh and natural foods** and whole-grain products. Avoid chemical preservatives and additives, artificial and imitation foods, refined and processed foods, and foods that are comprised of "nutritionally-empty calories."

Day 5 Recipe
<u>Frozen-Fish Dinner</u>

No recipe today. No cooking today. It's your day off! To find a frozen fish dinner, please go to Appendix A (page 198) which lists approximately 150 frozen dinners manufactured by Healthy Choice, Lean Cuisine and Smart Ones.

Perusing the list, it is obvious that there are not many frozen fish dinners for sale at supermarkets. Note that if you do not use all of the **340 Calories allocated for this Day 5 meal**, use the excess calories anyway you wish. Splurge on extra dessert or save the calories for the next day and have a larger piece of pizza!

Please read the important **Frozen-Food Safety Warning** in Appendix B on page 204.

<u>**Diet Tip of the Day:**</u> **Buy a pedometer** and start walking. For the average person 2,100 steps amounts to walking about one mile. A Harvard study has shown that 8,000 to 10,000 step per day promote weight loss. And you're not obliged to walk continuously until you accrue all 10,000 steps. Rather, all steps throughout the day to wherever and whenever count toward your daily total. Because 10000 steps a day may not be achievable by some people, particularly those who are elderly, sedentary, or who have chronic diseases, rather than insisting on a blanket 10000 steps per day, your initial stepping goal should your baseline steps plus an increment of an additional 2500 steps. (Your baseline being the number of steps you take in an average day.)

Day 6 Recipe

<u>Grandma's Pizza</u>

The following is a pizza recipe used by my Italian grandmother. She was from a small mountain village located between Rome and Naples.

Pizza dough: To save time use prepared dough, preferably whole wheat. Flour a large cutting board. <u>Divide one pound of prepared pizza dough into four parts</u>. Roll out each dough ball as thin as possible.

Tomato sauce: Sauté ½ small onion, chopped fine, in 1 tsp olive oil. Add two finely chopped garlic cloves, 1½ cups chopped plum tomatoes and ½ tsp chopped fresh oregano. Stir and cook about 5 minutes on a low flame.

Pizza preparation & cooking: On each pizza, spread evenly about ¼ cup of the tomato sauce. Add about ½ ounce of shredded part-skim mozzarella cheese, 1 tsp Parmesan cheese, 3 slices of a Portobello mushroom, some torn fresh basil, and drizzle with Evoo. Put pizzas on a pan and place in 475 ºF oven for about 15 to 20 minutes, or until crust is crisp and cheese is just melting. (Freeze left over sauce for use on Day 13.)

<u>Serves 4</u>.   Make four pizzas. Each pizza contains about 350 Calories.

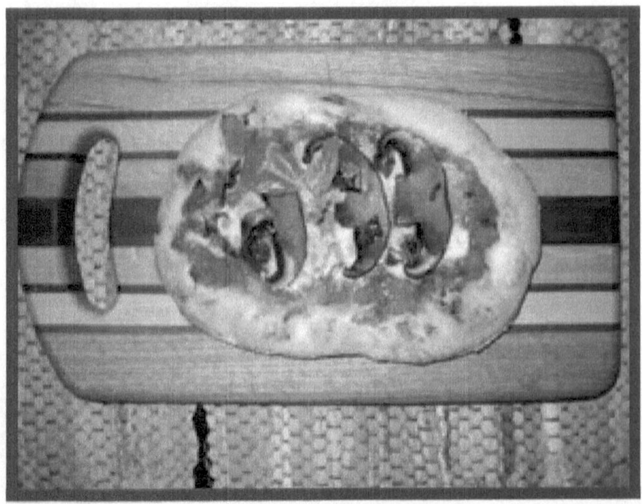

<u>Diet Tip of the Day:</u> For **life-long weight control** take a vigorous 30 to 60 minute walk everyday! That's right – everyday. Make exercise a nonflexible top priority part of your life. When it comes to exercise the key words are consistent, persistent, unyielding, dogged. Get the point?

Day 7 Recipe

<u>Chicken Dinner - Out</u>

No recipe today. No cooking today. Have a chicken dinner at your favorite restaurant, but make sure you choose a restaurant where you have a fighting chance to achieve your calorie goal. For 1200 Calorie meal plan, your goal for dinner is a **maximum of 580 Calories**. For 1500 Calorie meal plan, your goal for dinner is a **maximum of 630 Calories**. This includes appetizer, soup, main course, dessert and a glass of wine.

Tips for Eating Out: First, order simple, such as broiled chicken breast with steamed vegetables and brown rice. Tell the waiter you want no sauce, no gravy, nothing added. Then, knowing your calorie objective, and that chicken is about 50 Calories per ounce, most steamed vegetable servings average approximately 50 Calories per cup, and rice is about 100 Calories per ½ cup, decide how much to eat – and take the remainder home. If fresh fruit is not an option, pass on dessert and have the evening snack specified for that day in the diet.

In a restaurant, some nutritionists recommend you eat the low-calorie items on your plate first. Start with the salad, soup and veggies. By the time you get to the chicken and starches you will hopefully be full enough to be content with smaller portions of the higher-calorie choices.

Finally, some dieticians advise their dieting clients not to eat out. That's right. They believe eating at home is safer. But our thought is you have to eat out eventually so why not learn how while your resolve is high?

<u>**Diet Tip of the Day:**</u> When you're on a diet, eating in a restaurant can be a challenge, because most restaurant portions are huge, and can easily total more than 1,000 Calories. When eating in a restaurant decide how much to eat – and take the remainder home. A good general rule of thumb is to **eat half and bring the rest home**.

Day 8 Recipe
<u>Baked Salmon with Salsa</u>

This is a simple, straight-forward recipe. Again, the advantage of a simple recipe is there are no hidden calories.

    4 5 oz salmon fillets
    6 Tbsp bottled tomato-pepper salsa

Brown salmon fillets in non-stick pan and place in baking dish. Put fillets in an oven preheated to 350 ºF for about 10 minutes. Plate the salmon. Stir prepared tomato-pepper salsa and spoon it over the salmon.
<u>Serves 4</u>. One salmon fillet is about 215 Calories.

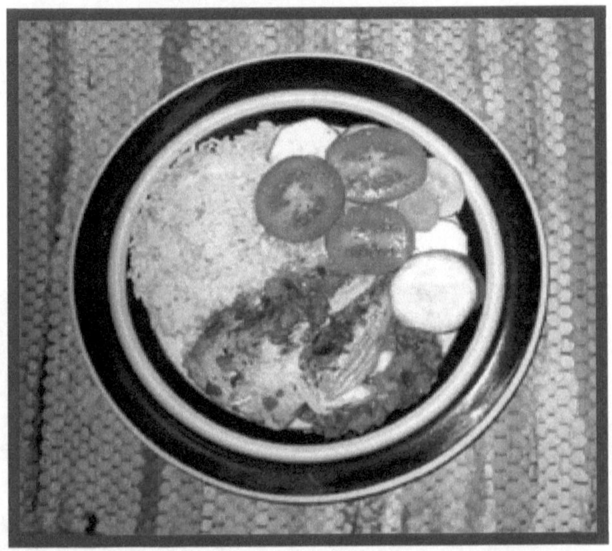

<u>**Diet Tip of the Day:**</u> **Have soup more often.** Most <u>non-cream-based</u> soups are filling and low-calorie.

Day 9 Recipe

<u>Veggie Burger</u>

Vegetable-based burgers can be purchased at your local supermarket. The patty of a veggie burger can be made from vegetables, soy, nuts, mushrooms, textured vegetable protein, dairy, or a combination of these foods.

Two popular veggie burgers are the Boca Burger and Gardenburger. The Boca Burger is made chiefly from soy protein and wheat gluten. (Boca Burger patties are 2.5 oz each and range from 60 to 90 Calories.) The original Gardenburger is made from mushrooms, onions, brown rice, rolled oats, cheese, and spices. (Gardenburger patties are 2.5 oz each and about 100 Calories.)

To prepare, follow package directions. The version shown below has an added slice of low-fat cheddar cheese. The lettuce, tomato and ketchup shown actually add very few extra calories.

The veggie burger patty plus low-fat cheese amounts to approximately 150 Calories. Add a seeded roll and the total rises to 290 Calories.

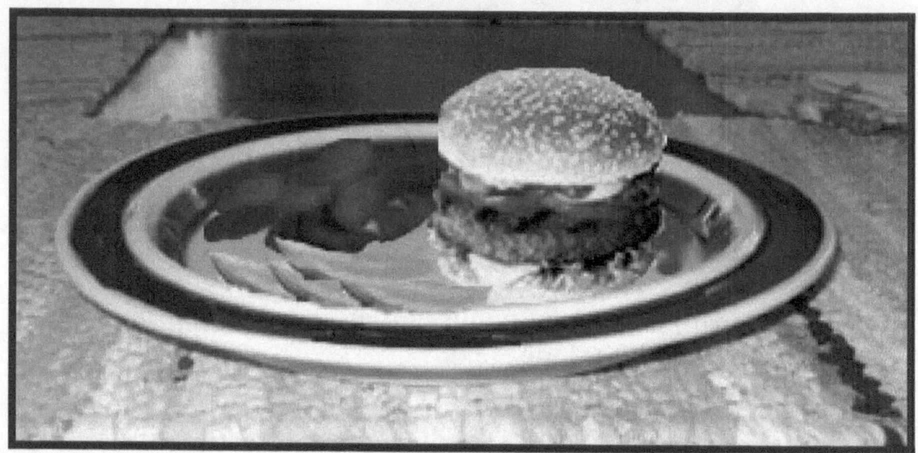

<u>Diet Tip of the Day:</u> Drink lots of water – about 8 glasses per day. Add a slice of lemon to make it more interesting. Often, when you think you're hungry, you are just thirsty. So, next time you head for a snack, drink some water first and see if that does it for you.

Day 10 Recipe

<u>Wild Blueberry Pancakes</u>

This recipe makes a relatively low calorie, wholesome batch of delicious wild blueberry-whole wheat-buttermilk pancakes.

  1 cup whole-wheat flour
  1 cup buttermilk
  1 egg
  1 Tbsp vegetable oil
  1 tsp baking powder
  ½ tsp baking soda

Stir ingredients until blended. Add ¾ cup blueberries and gently stir. Using medium heat, preheat a non-stick skillet coated with cooking spray. Pour slightly less than ¼ cup of batter onto skillet per pancake. Cook slowly until bubbles break on surface of pancake. Turn and cook until other side is lightly browned. Makes 8 pancakes.

Pictured below are wild-blueberry pancakes with two slices of turkey bacon.

<u>Serves 4</u>. Each pancake is about 95 Calories

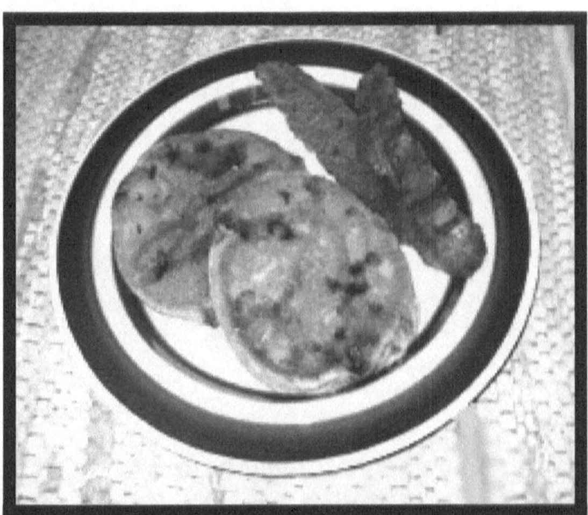

<u>Diet Tip of the Day:</u> A peanut butter sandwich on whole wheat bread with a glass of skim milk and an apple makes a nutritious, reasonably low-calorie lunch.

Day 11 Recipe

<u>Artichoke-Bean Salad</u>

1 can (19 oz) white kidney beans
10 artichoke hearts, quartered
⅓ cup chopped oregano
⅓ cup chopped parsley
3 cloves garlic, chopped
1 lemon, juiced

Combine ingredients in medium-size bowl. Stir in ¼ cup Evoo. Salt and black pepper to taste.

<u>Serves 6</u>. Artichoke-bean salad has approximately 190 Calories per serving.

Pictured on the plate below are two grilled chicken sausage links with salsa, steamed green beans and the artichoke-bean salad. Incidentally, this artichoke-bean combination over mixed salad greens served with a whole-grain bread makes a delicious, nutritious and reasonable low-calorie main course.

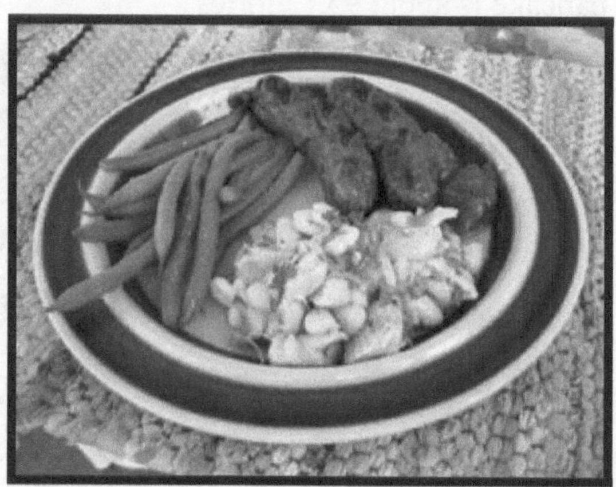

<u>Diet Tip of the Day:</u> Have a small meal before you go to a party. A hardboiled egg, an apple, and a thirst quencher (like water, tea, seltzer, or diet soda) will take the edge off your appetite and make it easier to resist the high-calorie goodies.

Day 12 Recipe

Fish Dinner - Out

No recipe today. No cooking today. Have a fish dinner at your favorite restaurant, but make sure you choose a restaurant where you have a good chance to achieve your calorie goal. For Day 12, your **goal for dinner is a maximum of 595 Calories**. This includes appetizer, soup, main course, dessert and a glass of wine.

Tips for Eating Out: The following is almost an exact repeat of advice given for Day 7. First, order simple, such as broiled fish with steamed vegetables and brown rice. Tell the waiter you want no sauce, no gravy, nothing added. Then, knowing your calorie objective, and that fish is about 50 Calories per ounce, most steamed vegetable servings average approximately 50 Calories per cup, and rice is about 100 Calories per ½ cup, decide how much to eat – and take the remainder home. If fresh fruit is not an option, pass on dessert and have the evening snack specified for that day in the diet.

In a restaurant, I recommend you eat the low-calorie items on your plate first. Start with the salad, soup and veggies. By the time you get to the fish and starches you will hopefully be full enough to be content with smaller portions of the higher-calorie choices.

Diet Tip of the Day: Phytonutrients are found in plant foods such as fruits, vegetables, whole grains, dried beans, nuts and seeds. Unlike protein, fat, vitamins and minerals, phytonutrients are not necessary for life, but evidence is growing that phytonutrients have many beneficial qualities.

Day 13 Recipe

<u>Pasta with Marinara Sauce</u>

Prepare the sauce as you did for the Day 6 pizza. But because the pizza sauce is a bit too thick, add ¼ cup of pasta liquid to thin it. (The spiral pasta shape shown below is called Fusilli, and is a favorite because all the ridges really hold the sauce.)

   ½ pound <u>whole-wheat</u> pasta

   ¼ tsp salt

Prepare the marinara tomato sauce as per Day 6 sauce but dilute it with ¼ cup of pasta liquid. Bring 2 quarts of lightly salted water to a boil. Add pasta and stir occasionally (to keep pasta from sticking to the bottom of the pot). Keep water boiling and cook until pasta are "al dente." (Cooking time is approximately 9 minutes.) Drain pasta, add marinara sauce and serve hot.

<u>Serves 4</u>. One serving is about 225 Calories.

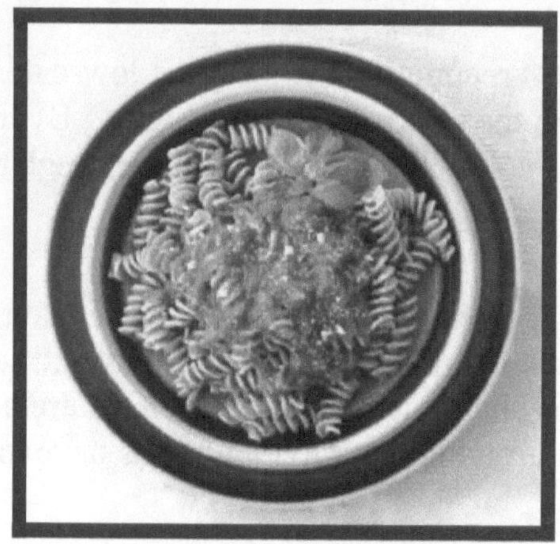

<u>Diet Tip of the Day:</u> **Beware of alcoholic beverages**. Beer has about 13 Calories per ounce, wine 25 Calories per ounce and whiskey 71 Calories per ounce.

Day 14 Recipe

"Oatena" Cereal Mix

Mixing nutritious cereals, hot or cold, is a good way to add variety as well as nutrition to a meal. This recipe features a mix of two whole grain cereals: Oatmeal and Wheatena.

   ⅓ cup Oatmeal
   ¼ cup (4 Tbsp) Wheatena
   ¾ cup water
   ½ cup skim milk
   ¼ cup blueberries
   10 raisins

Add Oatmeal, Wheatena, raisins and a dash of salt to a microwave-safe cereal bowl. Next add water and stir. Place bowl in microwave, on high power for about 1½ minutes, or until desired consistency is reached. The result is "Oatena," a mix of oatmeal and Wheatena, shown (half eaten) below.

Add skim milk and blueberries and serve hot. Because of the natural sugar in blueberries and raisins, adding sugar is not necessary.

Serves 1. About 310 Calories per serving

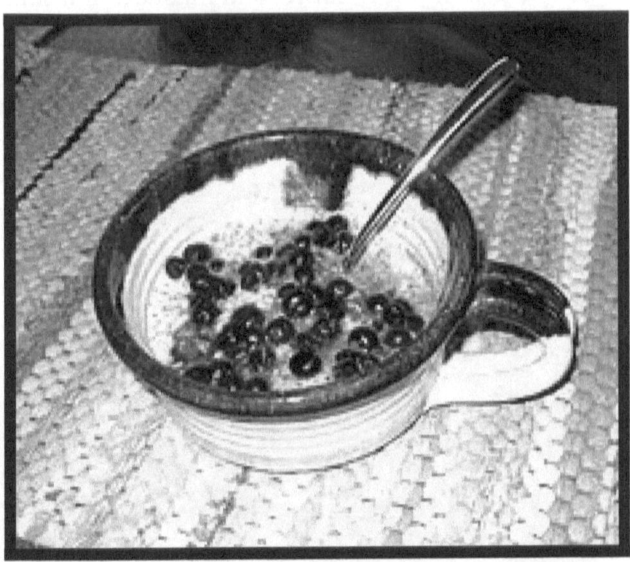

Diet Tip of the Day: Hot or cold cereal topped with fruit, and fat-free milk makes a nutritious, relatively low-calorie meal anytime.

Day 15 Recipe

<u>Tuna & Bean Salad</u>

- 1   tuna steak, about 2 inches thick (14 ounces)
- 2   tablespoons extra-virgin olive oil
- 1   tablespoon lemon juice
- 1   garlic clove, crushed
- 1   tablespoon Dijon mustard
- 1   15-ounce can cannellini beans, drained
- 1   small red onion, thinly sliced
- 2   red peppers, seeded and thinly sliced
- ½   cucumber, halved lengthwise and thinly sliced
- 6   cups watercress

Heat a ridged grill pan coated with cooking spray over medium-high heat. Season tuna steak on both sides with coarsely ground black pepper. Cook the tuna 4 minutes on each side - the outside should be browned and the center light pink. Be careful not to overcook. Remove from the pan and set aside.

Mix together the oil, lemon juice, garlic, and mustard in a salad bowl. Season with salt and pepper to taste. Add the cannellini beans, onion, peppers, cucumber and watercress. Toss gently to mix. Cut tuna into ½-inch thick slices. Arrange on top of salad and serve with lemon wedges. **<u>Serves 4</u>**. 355 Calories per serving

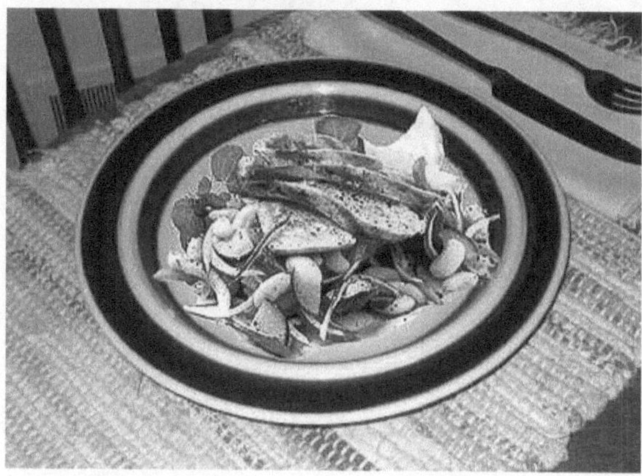

<u>Diet Tip of the Day:</u> In the United States, for a food to be labeled "**whole grain**" it must contain more than 51 percent whole grain by weight.

Day 16 Recipe

<u>Baked Red Snapper</u>

4 red snapper fillets – 4 oz each (salmon may be substituted)
½ cup white wine
½ cup non-fat yogurt mixed with half as much mustard
½ pound green beans
20 cherry tomatoes
4 tsp olive oil
1 cup wild rice, brown rice and wheat berry mix

Prepare rice mix per package directions.

Brown fillets in non-stick pan. Place fillets skin side down in baking dish coated with non-stick spray. Add white wine and cook in oven preheated to 350 ºF for about 15 minutes. Spoon pan juices over fillets. Salt and pepper to taste.

Place green beans in skillet. Add ¼-inch of water and cook over medium heat until water boils off. Add cherry tomatoes and olive oil. Stir well and sauté for a few minutes. Season with fresh rosemary and oregano. Salt and pepper to taste.

Plate red snapper fillet and spoon over yogurt-mustard sauce. Add green beans & tomato mix and the wild rice. Serve hot.

<u>Serves 4</u>. One plate consisting of one snapper fillet (215 Calories) with green beans & tomato mix (75 Calories) and wild rice (160 Calories) totals 450 Calories.

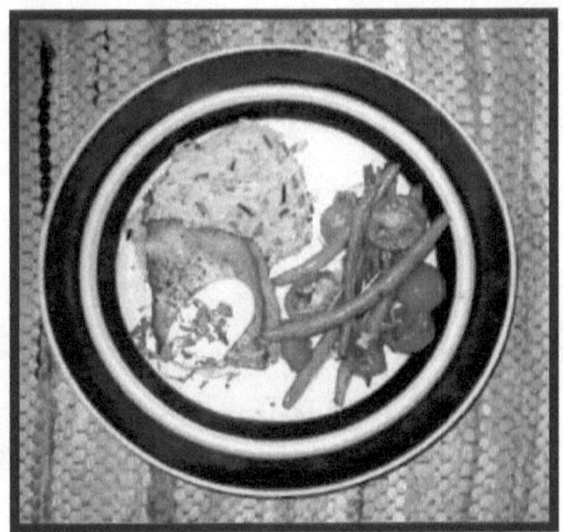

<u>Diet Tip of the Day:</u> **Don't have sweets in your house**. This makes them easier to resist. Out of sight, out of mind!

Day 17 Recipe

<u>Cajun Chicken Salad</u>

This is a perfect after-work, quick, nutritious and delicious dinner.

  4 boneless and skinless chicken breasts (about 5 oz each)
  1 bottle Cajun spices
  8 ounces mixed salad greens
  20 cherry tomatoes
  12 pitted black olives

Brush chicken breasts lightly with olive oil. Roll breasts in Cajun spices.
Brown breasts on non-stick oven-proof skillet. After breasts are brown,
put skillet in 350 ºF oven for approximately 15 minutes, or until done. Cut
breasts into ½-inch slices. (When the breasts are done, the meat should be
moist and white with no sign of pink.) Serve hot or keep in an oven or
warmer at 200 ºF until ready to plate.

Place chicken slices over a bed of mixed salad greens. Add tomatoes,
olives and 2 Tbsp of your favorite low-calorie salad dressing.

<u>Serves 4</u>. 330 Calories per serving.

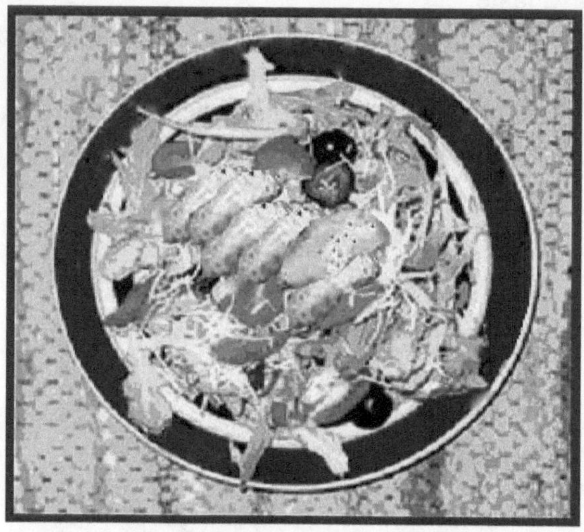

<u>Diet Tip of the Day:</u> Know that **fat-free isn't always your best bet**.
Very often sugar is substituted for fat and the calorie total remains the
same. Low fat does not necessarily mean low calorie! Rather, look for
low-calorie or reduced-calorie products.

Day 18 Recipe

<u>Grilled Swordfish</u>

1¼ pounds swordfish
1 bottle citrus-herb marinade
24 cherry tomatoes
4 medium potatoes
2 cups fresh spinach
1 tsp rosemary & juice of ¼ lemon
2 tsp extra virgin olive oil (Evoo)

Steam spinach with garlic and drizzle with Evoo. Cut up potatoes and place sprinkle with lemon juice, add rosemary, salt and black pepper. Place on grill for about 10 minutes, turning occasionally.

Toss cherry tomatoes in small amount Evoo. Add fresh oregano, salt and black pepper. Place on heavy-duty aluminum foil, seal and grill for about 3 minutes.

Marinade swordfish in citrus-herb vinaigrette. Grill on hot fire for about 5 minutes on one side and 3 minutes on the other, or until done as desired.

<u>Serves 4</u>. One plate consisting of grilled swordfish (250 Calories) with grilled potatoes (100 Calories) and cherry tomatoes (45 Calories) and steamed spinach (50 Calories) totals 445 Calories.

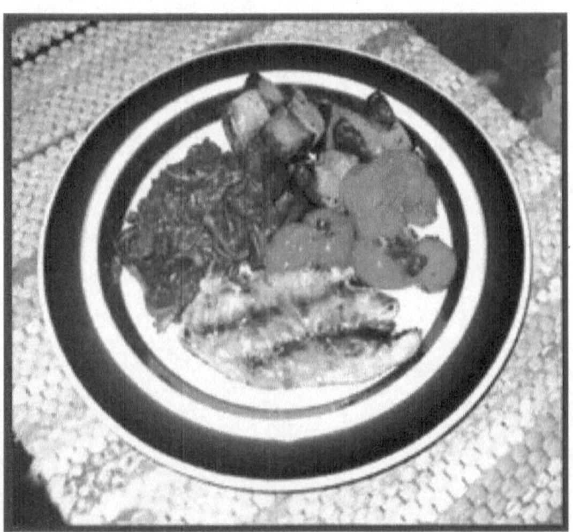

<u>Diet Tip of the Day:</u> Don't be in a hurry to lose weight. Slow weight loss is healthier, is more likely to be permanent, and is easier to sustain over the long haul.

Day 19 Recipe

<u>**Italian Food - Out**</u>

No recipe today. No cooking today. Have dinner at your favorite Italian restaurant, but make sure you choose a restaurant where you have a reasonable chance to achieve your calorie goal. For today, **your goal for dinner is a maximum of 640 Calories**. This includes any appetizer, soup, main course and a 4 ounce glass of wine.

Tips for Eating Italian: You can consume a lot of calories in an Italian restaurant – if you order carelessly. For example a typical portion is often loaded with about 1000 Calories, then add another 100 Calories for a glass of wine.

First rule, order simple. Look for a dish with lots of vegetables, some fish or chicken. Then, knowing your 640 Calorie objective, and that chicken and fish are about 50 Calories per ounce, most steamed vegetable servings average approximately 50 Calories per cup, and pasta is about 200 Calories per cup, decide how much of the meal you can eat – and take the remainder the diet. Also see Eating Out (page 13) for more guidance.

<u>Diet Tip of the Day</u>:   Another dilemma for dieters is **judging portion size**. It makes no sense to worry about whether to apportion 70 or 80 Calories per ounce for a cut of lean meat if you have no idea whether the portion you are planning to eat weighs four or ten ounces. To be successful, you must learn to estimate portion sizes with reasonable accuracy.

Day 20 Recipe

<u>Quick Pasta alla Puttanesca</u>

This famous pasta dish originated in Naples. Puttanesca means "ladies of the night." The exact origin of the name is unclear, but one thing is clear: It's delicious! Here is one of many recipe versions.

  ½ pound spaghetti (whole wheat preferred)
  20 black pitted olives
  1 can (14½ oz) diced tomatoes
  ½ can (4 oz) tomato sauce
  2 Tbsp Evoo
  3 cloves of garlic, chopped and 1Tbsp dried minced onion
  ½ tsp crushed red pepper flakes
  1 Tbsp capers drained and rinsed
  ¼ cup currants

Cook spaghetti according to package directions. Drain and return spaghetti to pot; add a teaspoon Evoo and toss to coat.
Heat 2 tablespoons olive oil in large skillet over medium-high heat. Add red pepper flakes; cook and stir 1 to 2 minutes or until sizzling. Add onion and garlic; cook and stir 1 minute. Finally, add tomatoes with juice, tomato sauce, olives, currants and capers. Cook over medium-high heat, stirring frequently, until sauce is heated through.
<u>Serves 4</u>. About 345 Calories per serving

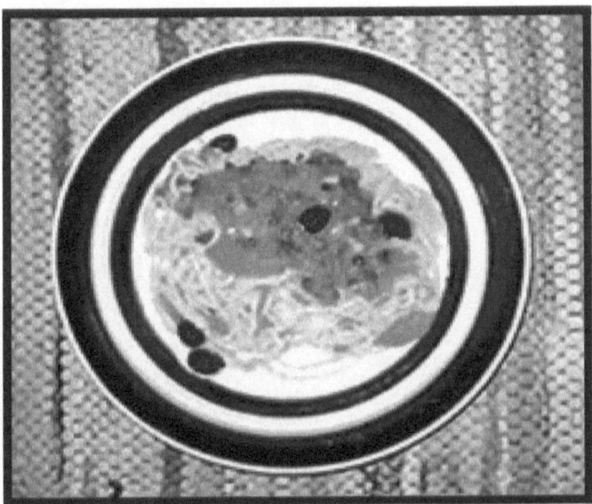

<u>Diet Tip of the Day:</u> Dilute juices, such as apple juice, orange, etc. with water. This cuts the flavor slightly but really reduces calorie content.

Day 21 Recipe

Frozen-Meat Dinner

No recipe today. No cooking today. It's your day off! To find a frozen meat dinner entrée please go to Appendix A (page 198) which lists approximately 150 frozen dinners manufactured by Healthy Choice, Lean Cuisine and Smart Ones.

Note that if you do not use all of the **300 Calories allocated for the Day 21 frozen dinner**, use the excess calories anyway you wish. Splurge on extra dessert or save the calories for another day.

Please read the important **Frozen-Food Safety Warning** in Appendix B on page 204.

Diet Tip of the Day: A good understanding of nutrition is not only vital for good health but also will help you control your weight over the long term. For example, did you know that foods that are an "excellent source" of a particular nutrient provide 20% or more of the Recommended Daily Value. Whereas, foods that are a "good source" of a nutrient provide between 10 and 20% of the Recommended Daily Value.

Day 22 Recipe

<u>Shrimp & Spinach Salad</u>

2 pounds shrimp in shell
½ pound small green beans, trimmed
½ pound baby spinach leaves
2 Tbsp lemon juice
¼ cup Evoo
2 tsp minced fresh dill
1 Tbsp minced green onion

To make vinaigrette, combine lemon juice, olive oil, dill, salt and pepper to taste and whisk until blended. Stir in minced onion and set aside.

Peel, de-vein and butterfly shrimp. Place shrimp in a bowl and add water to cover. Add 1 teaspoon of salt, and let stand for 10 minutes. Drain, rinse, drain again, and dry. Arrange shrimp in broiling pan without a rack. Brush shrimp with a little vinaigrette and place under preheated broiler, about 3 inches from heat. Broil about 3 to 4 minutes, turning shrimp once, or until both sides turn pink.

Remove shrimp from broiler and add remaining vinaigrette and green beans to the broiling pan. Stir to coat shrimp and beans with vinaigrette. Pour warm vinaigrette over spinach and toss quickly. Plate the spinach and arrange shrimp and green beans on top.

<u>Serves 4</u>. 310 Calories per serving.

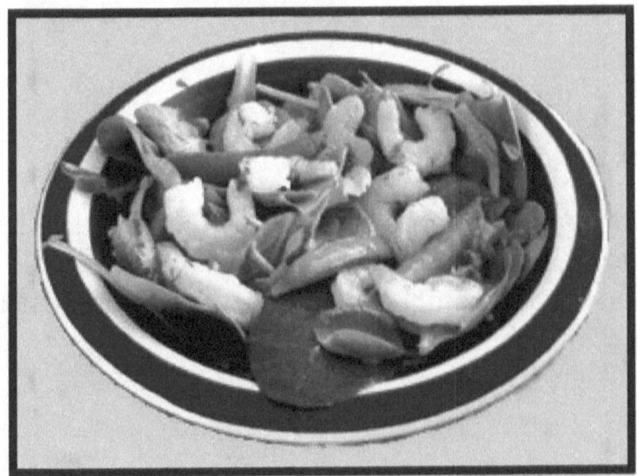

<u>Diet Tip of the Day:</u> After company leaves, have them take some of the leftover food (particularly the dessert) with them – or take the leftovers to work the next day.

Day 23 Recipe

<u>Beans & Greens Salad</u>

⅓ cup chopped oregano
⅓ cup chopped parsley
3 cloves garlic, chopped
1 lemon, juiced
Prepare salad dressing by combining above ingredients and stirring in ¼ cup Evoo. Salt and pepper to taste.
½ pound mesclun mix
¼ pound green beans
1 19 oz can garbanzo beans (chickpeas)
Arrange mesclun mix, garbanzo beans and green beans on a large platter.
Drizzle salad dressing over beans and greens.
<u>Serves 4</u>. Approximately 260 Calories per serving.

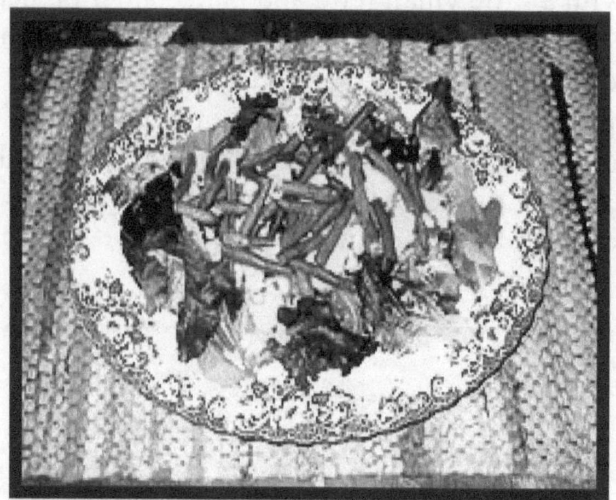

<u>Diet Tip of the Day:</u> Beans are a wonderful food but they are an incomplete protein. If however beans are eaten with a whole-grain bread, the combination forms a complete protein – just as complete and nutritious as meat, poultry, or fish.

Day 24 Recipe

<u>Four-Bean Plus Salad</u>

Note that the total caloric value of the salad will change very little, if the proportions of the bean varieties and corn are varied – according to taste.

- ½ cup canned red kidney beans, drained and rinsed
- ½ cup canned black beans, drained and rinsed
- ½ cup canned chick peas, drained and rinsed
- ½ cup canned cannelloni beans, drained and rinsed
- ½ cup canned corn, drained
- 1 small red pepper, chopped
- 1 small green pepper, chopped
- 2 Tbsp Evoo
- 2 Tbsp lemon juice

In a large bowl mix red kidney beans, black beans, chick peas, cannelloni beans, corn and chopped red and green peppers. Stir in Evoo and lemon juice and plate.

<u>Serves about 6</u>. One serving is ½ cup – with about 135 Calories per serving

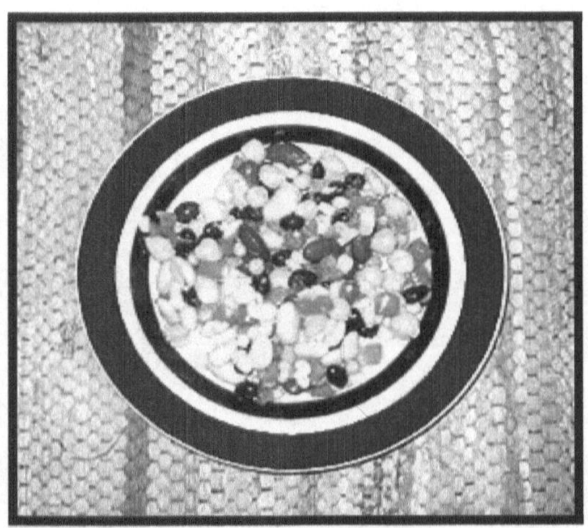

<u>Diet Tip of the Day:</u> Vigorous exercise doesn't necessarily stimulate you to overeat. Just the opposite. In many cases, exercise actually helps curb your appetite – immediately following a workout.

Day 25 Recipe

<u>Pan-Broiled Hanger Steak</u>

1¼ pounds hanger steak, well trimmed of fat
¼ cup lime juice
8 small new potatoes, peeled and halved
12 cherry tomatoes, cut in half

Season both sides of steak with salt and pepper and place in sealable plastic bag with lime juice. Refrigerate for about one hour.

Boil potatoes about 10 minutes. Rinse in cold water. Sauté potatoes in small amount of vegetable oil over medium-high heat until brown.

Sauté cherry tomatoes in small amount of olive oil over medium-high heat until skin begins to crack. Season with chopped fresh basil.

Heat a skillet over medium-high heat. Sear hanger steak on one side for about 5 minutes. Turn over and sear other side approximately 5 minutes (for medium done). Pour off any fat that may have accumulated. Carve into ½-inch slices.

<u>Serves 4.</u> About 320 Calories per serving (for the hanger steak only)

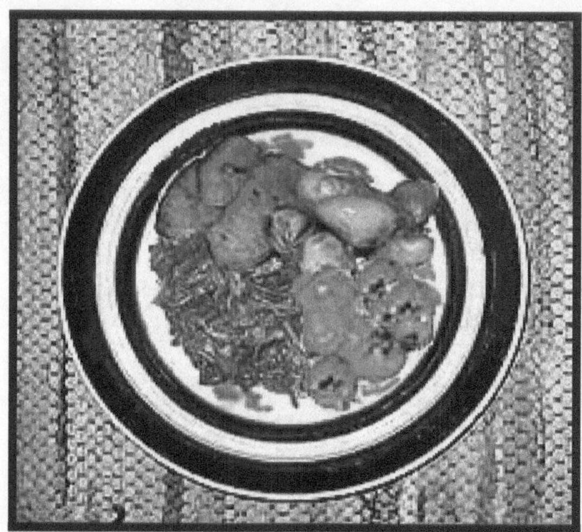

<u>Diet Tip of the Day:</u> If you find yourself at a party, don't stand near the food! Be aware of the temptation. Make the effort, and you'll find you eat less.

Day 26 Recipe

<u>Grilled Scallops and Polenta</u>

1 pound sea scallops
¾ cup polenta cornmeal
¾ cup skim milk
1 medium Portobello mushroom
½ pound green beans
¼ cup chopped red onion
16 asparagus spear
1 tsp Evoo

Bring 1½ cups of water and skim milk to rapid boil. Add salt to taste and slowly add polenta while stirring. Reduce heat. Continue stirring until desired consistency is reached. Pour polenta into lightly greased pan. After polenta has cooled cover and refrigerate. Cut chilled polenta into 4 pieces. Grill on medium-hot fire – about two minutes on each side.
Brush Portobello mushroom and asparagus spear with Evoo and place on grill for about 3 minutes on each side.
Grill scallops on medium-hot fire. Turn after two minutes or when first side turns opaque. Grill until second side turns opaque – about another 2 minutes. Don't overcook but test a scallop by cutting to make sure it's cooked through. Salt and pepper to taste.
<u>Serves 4</u>. The food on the plate pictured below totals 380 Calories.

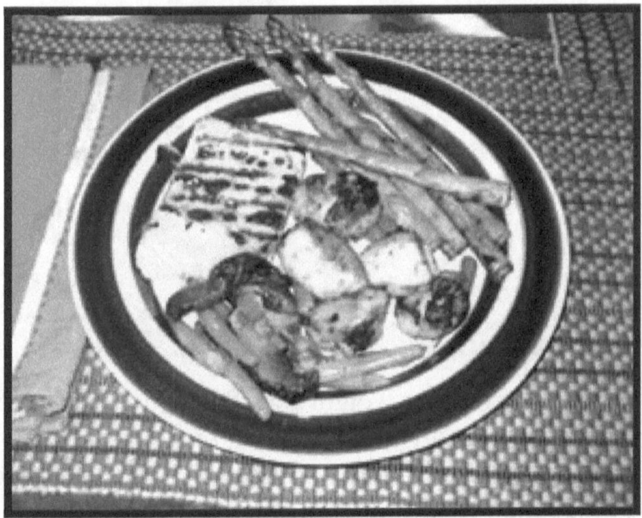

<u>Diet Tip of the Day:</u> To have better control of what you eat **bring your lunch to work**.

Day 27 Recipe

Fettuccine in Summer Sauce

This sauce is often served in the summer because it's lighter than what is usually dished up with pasta. But despite its name the sauce is wonderful year round.

  ½ pound fettuccine

  8 ounces fresh asparagus, trimmed & cut into 2" pieces

  20 cherry tomatoes, halved

  2 Tbsp plus 1 tsp Evoo

  2 cloves of garlic, chopped

  ½ small onion, diced

Cook fettuccine according to package directions. Drain and return pasta to pot; add a teaspoon Evoo and toss to coat. Meanwhile steam asparagus and drain.

In large skillet over medium-high heat, sauté cherry tomatoes in 2 Tbsp olive oil until skin begins to crack. Add onion and cook until translucent. Stir in garlic . Thin sauce with pasta liquid to desired consistency. Toss cooked pasta and asparagus into sauce and serve immediately.

Serves 4. About 290 Calories per serving

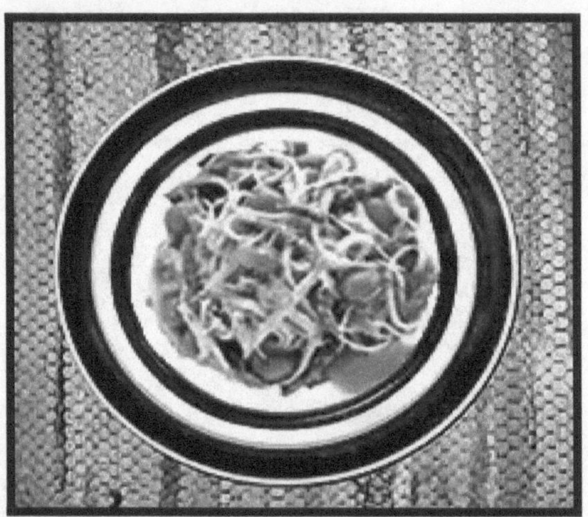

Diet Tip of the Day: A major weight-loss fallacy is that you can get rid of abdominal fat by working your abdominal muscles. This is based on the incorrect belief that fat is eliminated from a particular part of your body if you engage the muscles underneath that layer of fat. No such luck.

Day 28 Recipe
<u>Frozen Chicken Meal</u>

No recipe today. No cooking today. It's your day off! To find a frozen chicken dinner entrée please go to Appendix A (page 198) which lists approximately 150 frozen dinners manufactured by Healthy Choice, Lean Cuisine and Smart Ones.

Note that if you do not use all of the **300 Calories allocated for the Day 28 frozen dinner**, use the excess calories anyway you wish. Splurge on extra dessert or save the calories for another day.

Please read the important **Frozen-Food Safety Warning** in Appendix B on page 204.

<u>**Diet Tip of the Day:**</u>   The **general weight-change rule is "last on first off."** Assume as you gained weight, the first place you noticed it was on your thighs, next your buttocks, then your face. As you lose weight, it generally will come off in the reverse order, first from your face, then your rear and finally your thighs. And there is not much you can do about that. The truth is there is no food, no exercise, no magic belt, and no pill that will cause your body to lose fat in one place rather than another.

Day 29 Recipe

<u>Barbequed Shrimp</u>

1½ pounds large shrimp
3 Tbsp bottled barbeque sauce
4 medium ears of corn

Pour barbeque sauce into shallow bowl. Toss shrimp in barbeque sauce to coat. Place shrimp on medium-hot grill. Turn shrimp after about two minutes or when shrimp turn pink. Grill until second side turns pink – approximately another 2 minutes. Don't overcook but test a shrimp by cutting to make sure it is cooked through. Salt and pepper to taste. Serve hot or at room temperature.

<u>Serves 4</u>. About 160 Calories per serving (shrimp only).

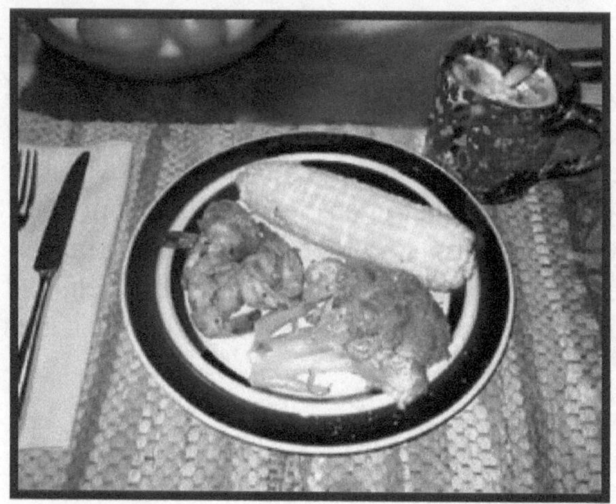

<u>Diet Tip of the Day:</u> A very important weight-profile parameter is your waist-to-hip ratio. Health risks for heart attack and stroke increase considerably for men with a ratio above 1.0 and for women with a ratio above 0.8. To calculate your ratio, measure your waist size (at its narrowest circumference) and divide it by your hip size (at the widest wedge).

Day 30 Recipe

Pasta e Fagioli

This is one variation of a traditional, nutritious peasant dish served in
Italy.

14.5-oz can whole tomatoes with juice, crushed
14.5-oz can cannellini beans, drained
1   cup of any tube-shaped pasta
2   tablespoon olive oil
1   medium onion, diced
2   cloves garlic, minced
1   stalk celery, finely chopped
3   cups chicken stock
2   cups fresh baby spinach or escarole
1   tsp dried basil
½   teaspoon dried oregano
2   Tbsp fresh parsley, chopped

Heat olive oil, onion and celery in large saucepan over medium heat.
Sauté until onions are golden brown. Add garlic and stir constantly for
one minute. Pour in tomatoes and their juices and bring to a boil. Add
beans and chicken stock and return to a boil. Stir in spinach (or escarole)
and seasonings. Simmer for about 5 minutes. Add pasta and cook about
15 minutes or until pasta is tender but firm. If needed, thin soup with hot
water. Ladle into soup bowls. Garnish with grated Parmesan cheese. Salt
and pepper to taste.

Serves 4. About 300 Calories per serving.

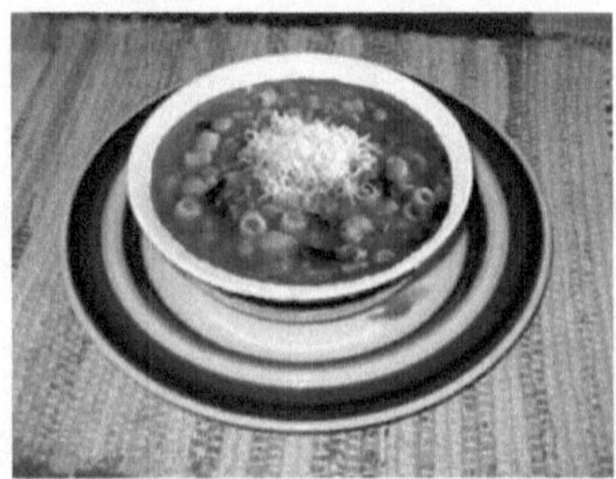

Diet Tip of the Day: Pasta alone is an incomplete protein. But when
combined with beans, a complete protein results – that is a protein that
contains all eight essential amino acids.   The dish is every bit as nutritious
as meat, fish or poultry.

Day 31 - Recipe

Tina's Baked Sea Bass

  4 4-ounce Chilean sea bass fillets
  ½ pound green beans
  ¾ pint cherry tomatoes (about 20)
  ¾ cup brown rice (prepare per package directions)

<u>Sea Bass:</u> Dust filets with flour. Dip in egg wash & then Panko bread crumbs. Place fillets in baking dish coated with non-stick spray. Bake about 15 minutes in oven preheated to 350 ºF.

<u>Green Beans & Tomato:</u> Place green beans in skillet. Add ¼-inch of water and cook over medium heat until water boils off. Add cherry tomatoes and olive oil. Stir well and sauté for a few minutes. Season with fresh rosemary and oregano.

<u>Brown Rice-Pesto mix:</u> Prepare brown rice per package directions. Add 4 teaspoons packaged "green" pesto. Mix thoroughly.

<u>Red Pepper Sauce:</u> Blend one roasted red pepper (skinned), ½ cup non-fat yogurt, 1 tsp lemon juice, 1 Tbsp olive oil, 1 Tbsp chili sauce, and a dash of Worcestershire sauce.

<u>Serves 4</u>. One plate consisting of one sea bass fillet with spooned over red pepper sauce (150 Calories), green beans & tomato mix (75 Calories), brown rice-pesto mix (120 Calories) and half ear of corn (50 Calories) – totals about 395 Calories.

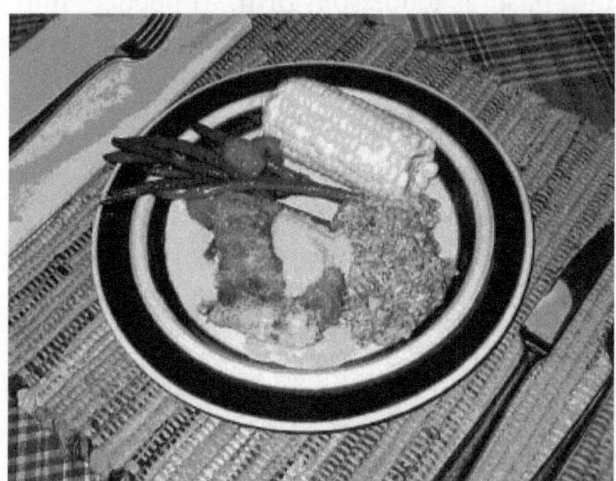

<u>**Diet Tip of the Day:**</u> Protein foods make you **feel full longer** and help prevent overeating.

<h1 style="text-align:center">Day 32 - Recipe</h1>

<u>Turkey Tenders & Vegetables</u>

 2   turkey breast tenderloins (about 1½ lb)
 1   medium eggplant (about ¾ lb)
 ¾   pound yellow (summer) squash
 2   medium plum tomatoes, quartered

<u>Marinade</u>: Whisk in a bowl 2 tsp lemon zest, ¼ cup lemon juice, 2 Tbsp olive oil, 1 Tbsp chopped garlic, 1 Tbsp chopped rosemary, ¼ tsp salt and a pinch of black pepper. Put marinade and turkey breasts in large re-sealable plastic bag. Refrigerate about 45 minutes

Slice eggplant and squash lengthwise about ½-inch thick. Place with tomatoes on a baking sheet coated with a nonstick spray.

Grill turkey breasts approximately 7 to 9 minutes per side, or until an instant-read thermometer inserted from the side to middle registers 160°F. Slice turkey and set aside.

Grill eggplant and zucchini about 4 minutes per side, or until just tender. Grill tomatoes about 2 minutes per side, or until charred but not soft. Cut vegetables bite-size and toss with remaining marinade. Serve with sliced turkey.

<u>**Serves 4**</u>. About 350 Calories per serving (includes turkey and veggies)

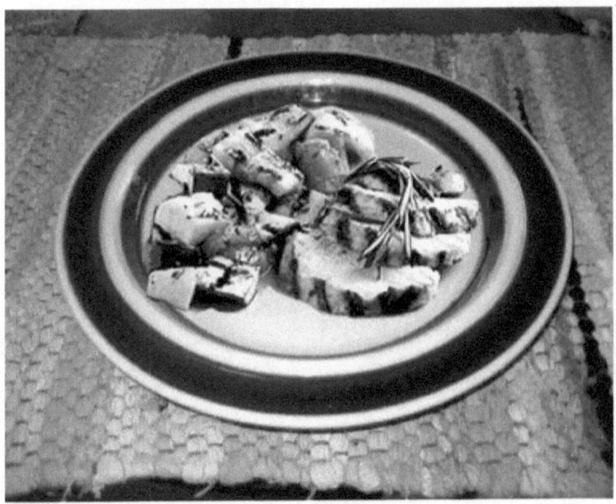

<u>**Diet Tip of the Day:**</u> It's a lot easier to eat 1,000 Calories than it is to burn 1,000 Calories exercising. So a stroll after dinner isn't going to offset the calories you ingested eating a Big Mac plus fries.

Day 33 - Recipe

Frozen-Fish Dinner

No recipe today. No cooking today. It's your day off! To find a frozen fish dinner, please go to Appendix A (page 198) which lists approximately 150 frozen dinners manufactured by Healthy Choice, Lean Cuisine and Smart Ones.

Perusing the list, it is obvious that there are not many frozen fish dinners for sale at supermarkets. Note that if you do not use all of the **340 Calories allocated for this Day 5 meal**, use the excess calories anyway you wish. Splurge on extra dessert or save the calories for the next day and have a larger piece of pizza!

Please read the important **Frozen-Food Safety Warning** in Appendix B on page 204

Diet Tip of the Day: It's amazing how many people tend to confuse thirst with hunger. This often results in overeating when actually drinking water might be the solution. So, the next time you have a seemingly uncontrollable food craving, try drinking a glass of water instead.

Day 34 - Recipe

Pasta Rapini

  2 cloves garlic - coarsely chopped
  1½ cups of crushed San Marzano tomatoes
  2 cups Rapini (broccoli rabe)
  1 tablespoon crushed red pepper flakes (optional)
  ½ pound medium-sized whole wheat pasta

<u>Tomato Sauce:</u> In large pan, sauté two tablespoons olive oil over medium-high heat. Add the garlic and sauté until translucent (but not browned). Add crushed San Marzano tomatoes (use plum tomatoes if San Marzano are not available) and bring to a boil. Reduce heat to low and simmer for about 30 minutes or until cooked. Season with salt and pepper. Set aside.

<u>Rapini:</u> Discard the tough stems and slice into 2-inch pieces. Bring a pot of water to a boil. Add Rapini (a variety of the vegetable broccoli rabe) and 1 tablespoon salt. Blanch Rapini about 5 minutes or until slightly cooked but still crunchy at stems. Drain, set aside and cover.

Cook pasta according to package instructions until al dente. Three minutes before pasta is ready, add the Rapini to the sauté pan (containing the tomato sauce). Heat mixture over medium heat. Drain pasta and add it to the pan with the Rapini and tomatoes. Add hot pepper flakes (optional) and toss for 1 to 2 minutes over high heat. Drizzle lightly with extra virgin olive oil and plate. Delicious!

Serves 4. About 290 Calories per serving

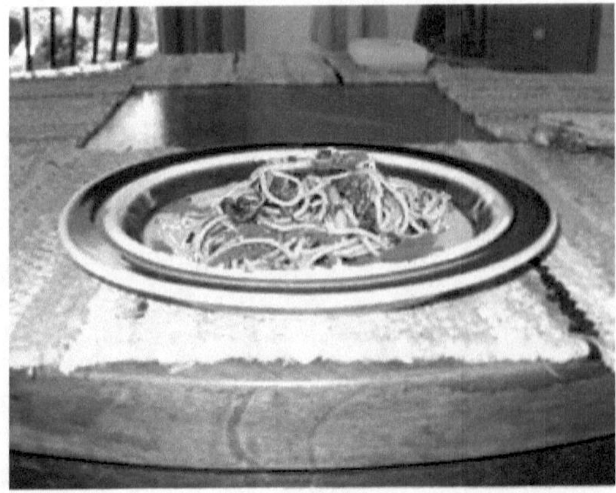

<u>Diet Tip of the Day:</u> Keep a daily food log to **record everything you eat**. For some people it really works wonders.

<u>Chicken Dinner - Out</u>

No recipe today. No cooking today. Have a chicken dinner at your favorite restaurant, but make sure you choose a restaurant where you have a fighting chance to achieve your calorie goal. For your chicken dinner out, your maximum allowable calories (includes appetizer, soup, main course and dessert) are as follows:

- For the **1,200 Calorie Diet**: 530 Calories
- For the **1,500 Calorie Diet**: 630 Calories

Tips for Eating Chicken Out: First, order simple and order skinless white meat only, such as broiled chicken breast with steamed vegetables and brown rice. (Incidentally, feel free to substitute skinless white meat turkey for chicken.) Tell the waiter you want no sauce, no gravy, nothing added. Then, knowing your calorie objective, and that chicken is about 50 Calories per ounce, most steamed vegetable servings average approximately 50 Calories per cup, and rice is about 100 Calories per ½ cup, decide how much to eat – and take the remainder home. If fresh fruit is not an option, pass on dessert and have the evening snack specified for that day in this diet.

In a restaurant, some nutritionists recommend you eat the low-calorie items on your plate first. Start with the salad, soup and veggies. By the time you get to the chicken and starches you will hopefully be full enough to be content with smaller portions of the higher-calorie choices.

Finally, some dieticians advise their dieting clients not to eat out. That's right. They believe eating at home is safer. But our thought is you have to eat out eventually so why not learn how while your resolve is high?

<u>Diet Tip of the Day</u>: To determine your frame size, circle your wrist with your thumb and third finger. If the tips of your fingers overlap, you have a small frame. If they just touch you are medium, and if they don't touch you have a large frame.

<u>Grilled Tilapia</u>

Tilapia is a mild, white fish that inhabits fresh water. This fish has very low levels of mercury because it's fast-growing, short-lived, and mostly eats a vegetarian diet. According to the Monterey Bay Aquarium, choose tilapia farmed in the U.S., in environmentally friendly systems. "Avoid" farmed tilapia from China and Taiwan, where pollution and weak management are a problem.

   4 Tilapia filets (about 6 ounces each)

<u>Marinade:</u> ¾ cup olive oil, ½ lemon, juiced, 1 tablespoons oregano, ½ teaspoon black pepper, ¼ cup red wine vinegar, ½ cup finely chopped parsley, 2 cloves garlic, minced and 2 dashes Tabasco (optional).

Combine all ingredients (except filets) in a large re-sealable plastic bag and shake well. Then place fish filets in the marinade for 30 minutes. Remove fillets from marinade and cook on hot grill for approximately 2 to 3 minutes per side.

<u>Serves 4.</u> About 300 Calories per serving (fish only)

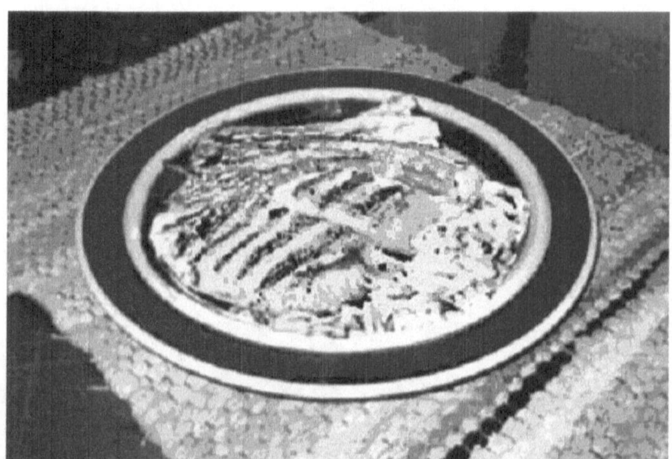

Photo shows two fish filets. Diet serving size is <u>one filet</u>.

<u>Diet Tip of the Day:</u> One serving of asparagus can provide you with 66% of your daily folate needs. Folate is a B-vitamin which is involved with cellular division, and therefore aids the development of a baby's nervous system.

Crab Cakes

- 1 lb jumbo crab meat
- 1½ Tbsp light mayonnaise
- 1½ Tbsp chopped green bell pepper
- 2 medium green onions, chopped
- 1 large egg, beaten
- 1 cup panko bread crumbs
- 2 Tbsp canola oil
- ¼ tsp black pepper

Drain crab meat on layers of paper towels. Combine crab meat, bell pepper, mayonnaise, black pepper, onions and egg. Stir in ¼ cup panko bread crumbs. (Place remaining panko in shallow dish.)

Divide crab meat mixture into 8 portions. Shape portions into ¾-inch thick patties and dredge in panko. Place non-stick skillet over medium heat and add 1 Tbsp oil. Add dredged patties and cook 3 minutes on each side or until golden.

Prepare remoulade: Combine ¼ cup light mayonnaise, 2 tsp minced shallots, 1 tsp chopped tarragon, 1 tsp chopped parsley, 1½ tsp Dijon mustard and ¾ tsp wine vinegar. Serve remoulade with crab cakes.
Serves 4. 320 Calories per serving (2 crab cakes)

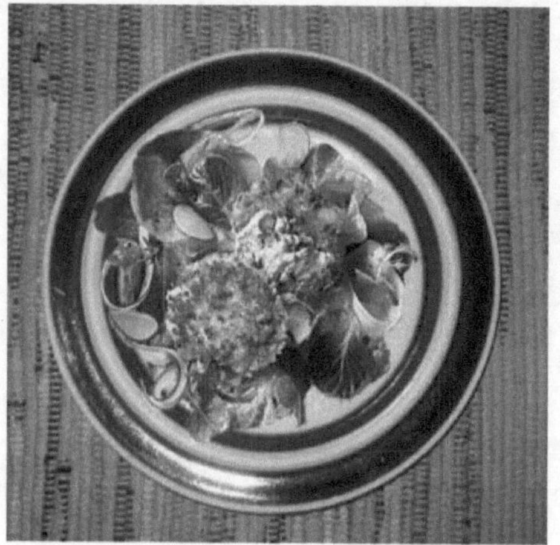

Diet Tip of the Day: **Understanding nutrition** is not only vital for good health but also will help you control your weight over the long term.

<u>Pan-Broiled Lamb Chop</u>

Pan broiling is a quick, easy and a relatively low-calorie technique that can be used to cook many meats.

Start with a rib lamb chop about ¾-inch thick that weighs roughly 6 ounces. Next, it is very important to carefully trim all the visible fat. (After removing the fat and accounting for the bone, about 4 ounces of lean meat should remain.)

Season the chop with salt and ground black pepper. Heat a well-seasoned cast iron or nonstick skillet over high heat. Add the chop (or chops) and cook approximately 4 minutes on each side. (Check center of chop with a small incision to determine when the meat is done.)   Plate and serve immediately.

<u>Serves 1</u>: About 320 Calories per chop

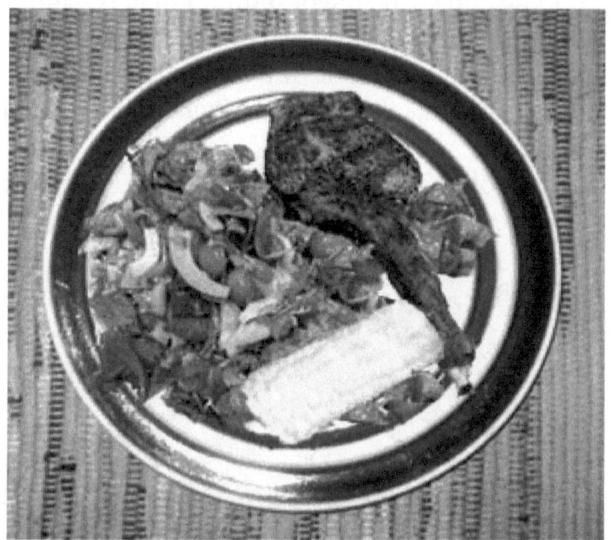

Note corn-on-the-cob is only for the 1,800-Calorie diet.

<u>**Diet Tip of the Day:**</u> According to a study published in the Journal of Food Chemistry, broccoli, spinach, kale, Brussels sprouts and other dark green vegetables have the highest cancer-fighting potential found in produce.

Day 39 - Recipe

<u>Chicken with Veggies</u>

  4 boneless, skinless chicken breast halves (about 5 oz each)
12 broccoli florets
  1 bunch of asparagus
  2 ripe medium-size tomatoes
  2 tablespoons Lo-Cal (light) salad dressing

Place evenly cut broccoli and asparagus spears in a microwave-safe pan, add a little water to bottom of the pan and top with microwave-safe plastic wrap. (Be sure to pull back one corner of the plastic topper so some steam can escape.) Check veggies periodically and take them out of the microwave when they reach desired softness.

Season chicken breasts evenly with salt and pepper. Heat a large nonstick skillet over medium-high heat. Coat pan with cooking spray. Cook chicken about 4 minutes on each side or until no pink remains.

For each serving, plate one chicken breast and a portion of the steamed broccoli and asparagus. Add one-half of a tomato cut into pieces. Drizzle about 2 tablespoons of a light salad dressing that contains no more than 50 Calories in 2 tablespoons.

<u>Serves 4</u>: One serving of chicken breast halve, veggies & dressing is about 365 Calories.

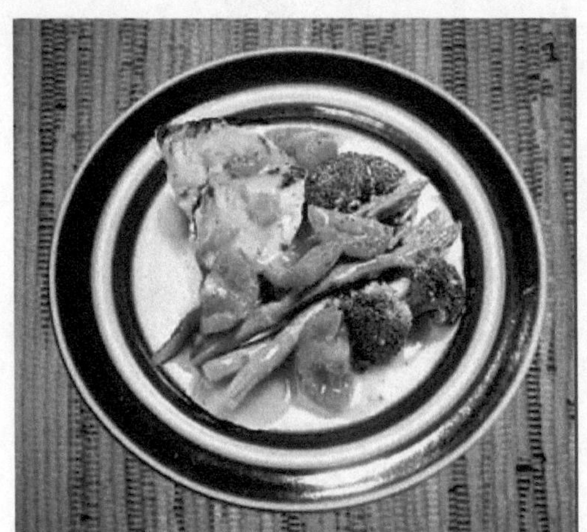

Shown drizzled with Light Thousand Island dressing.

<u>Diet Tip of the Day:</u> Steaming in a microwave oven is one of the best ways to cook veggies so they retain nutrients. Another advantage is the cooking adds no fat or sodium.

<u>Fish Dinner - Out</u>

No recipe today. No cooking today. Have a fish dinner at your favorite restaurant, but make sure you choose a restaurant where you have a good chance to achieve your calorie goal. For today, your **goal for dinner is a maximum of 595 Calories**. This includes appetizer, soup, main course and dessert.

Tips for Eating Fish Out: The following is almost an exact repeat of the advice given eating out on previous days. First, order simple, such as broiled fish with steamed vegetables and brown rice. Tell the waiter you want no sauce, no gravy, nothing added. Then, knowing your calorie objective, and that fish is about 50 Calories per ounce, most steamed vegetable servings average approximately 50 Calories per cup, and rice is about 100 Calories per ½ cup, decide how much to eat – and take the remainder home. If fresh fruit is not an option, pass on dessert and have the evening snack specified for that day in the diet.

In a restaurant, some nutritionists recommend you eat the low-calorie items on your plate first. Start with the salad, soup and veggies. By the time you get to the fish and starches you will hopefully be full enough to be content with smaller portions of the higher-calorie choices.

<u>Diet Tip of the Day:</u> For **life-long weight control** take a vigorous 30 to 60 minute walk everyday! That's right – everyday. Make exercise a nonflexible top priority part of your life. When it comes to exercise the key words are consistent, persistent, unyielding, dogged. Get the point?

Day 41 - Recipe

<u>Tina's Healthy Frittata</u>

- 3 large eggs, plus 3 egg whites
- ¾ cup reduced-fat cottage cheese
- 4 ounces smoked gouda cheese, shredded (about 1 cup)
- 1 teaspoon minced fresh rosemary
- 3 cloves garlic, thinly sliced
- 2 tablespoons Evoo
- 1 medium onion, chopped
- 16-ounce package frozen mixed vegetables, thawed
- 2 tablespoons grated parmesan cheese
- 1 scant teaspoon paprika

Position a rack in the upper third of your oven and preheat to 450 degrees F. Whisk eggs and egg whites in a bowl. Add the cottage cheese and whisk until almost smooth. Whisk in the gouda and rosemary. In a 10-inch nonstick skillet over medium-high, cook the garlic in the olive oil. Heat until garlic starts to brown, about 1 to 2 minutes. Add onion, season with salt and cook 2 minutes. Add the vegetables, increase the heat to high and cook until just tender, about 5 minutes. Reduce the heat to medium.

Spread the egg mixture evenly in the pan. Cook, without disturbing until a thin crust forms on the bottom, about 2 minutes. Run a rubber spatula around the edge to release egg from the pan. Continue cooking until the bottom is golden, about 2 to 3 minutes. Sprinkle with the parmesan and paprika. Transfer skillet to the oven and bake about 5 to 7 minutes. Remove from the oven, cover and let sit, 5 to 7 minutes. Cut into 4 wedges.
<u>Serves 4</u>. 320 Calories per serving (¼ of frittata)

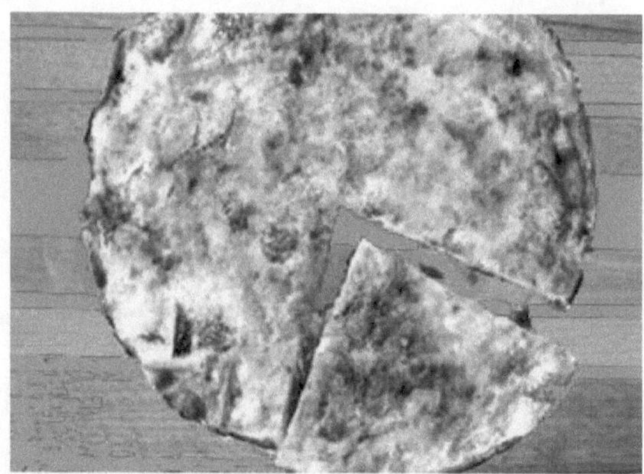

Photo shows frittata on cutting board - hot from skillet.

Day 42 - Recipe

<u>Dawn's Blueberry Muffins</u>

Wholesome whole-wheat blueberry muffins just like grandma used to make.
Serve them at breakfast, or as a nutritious dessert, or a wonderful snack.
(Make a dozen. Have one today and store the remainder in your freezer until
they are called for again later in the diet.)

    4 ounces bran flakes
    ¼ cup sugar
    1¼ cups whole wheat flour
    1 teaspoon baking soda
    ¼ teaspoon baking powder
    ¼ teaspoon salt
    ½ cup blueberries (fresh or frozen)
    1 egg, beaten
    1 cup buttermilk
    ¼ cup vegetable oil

Preheat oven to 400 °F. Coat muffin tins with nonstick cooking spray. In a
bowl combine dry ingredients. In another bowl combine wet ingredients and
mix thoroughly. Add wet ingredients to dry ingredients and mix until just
blended. Do not over mix. Gently fold in blueberries. Spoon batter into
muffin tins until two-thirds full. Bake 15 minutes or until muffin tops are
golden brown.

<u>**Yield**</u> is 12 Muffins, 145 Calories each

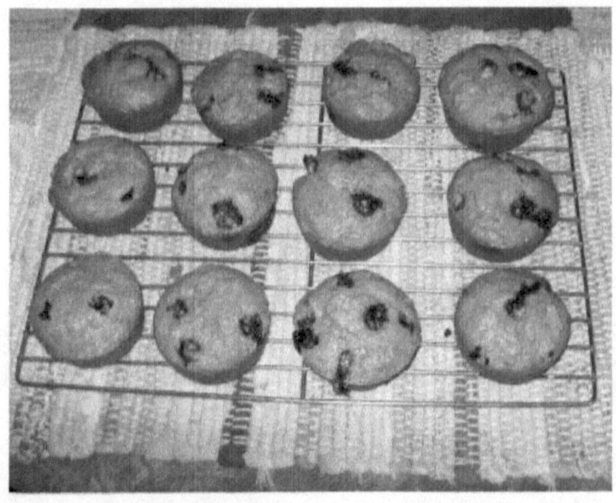

<u>**Diet Tip of the Day:**</u> **Acquire a good low-calorie cookbook**. Be sure the
recipes cover breakfast, lunch and dinner, and all the recipes contain
nutritional information, especially the calories per serving.

Day 43 - Recipe

Beef Kebob

  1 lb boneless beef tenderloin steaks, 1" thick
  8 ounces medium mushrooms
  2 medium bell peppers (any color), cut in pieces
Marinate ingredients:
  2 tablespoons olive oil
  1 tablespoon chopped fresh oregano
  2 cloves garlic, minced
  ½ teaspoon ground black pepper

Cut beef steak into 1-inch square pieces. Combine marinate ingredients in large bowl. Add beef, mushrooms and bell pepper pieces. Toss to coat. Cover bowl and refrigerate for about two hours. Thread beef and vegetable pieces onto eight 12-inch metal skewers.

Grill kebobs over medium-high heat for 8 to 10 minutes, turning occasionally. Check center of meat with a small incision to determine when the meat is done.

Microwave a one-pound package of frozen mixed vegetables. Plate two kebob skewers and about one-quarter of the mixed veggies.
Serves 4. One plate consisting of two kebob skewers (350 Calories) plus ¼ pound of mixed green vegetables (40 Calories) totals about 390 Calories.

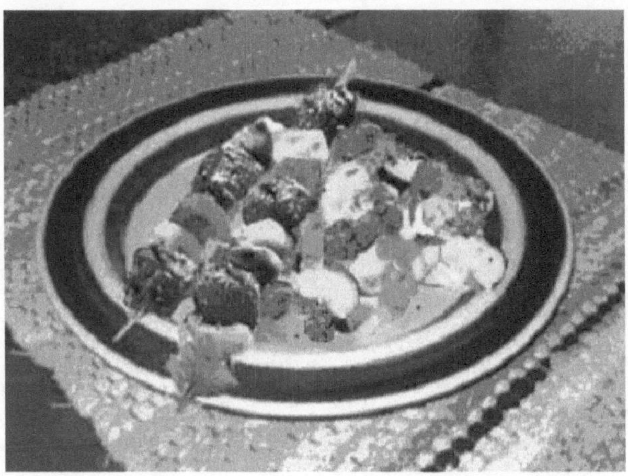

<u>**Diet Tip of the Day**</u>: Remember your stomach is about the size of your fist. So it doesn't take much food to fill it comfortably.

<h1 style="text-align:center">Day 44 - Recipe</h1>

<u>Baked Haddock</u>

- 4 4-oz haddock fillets (or salmon fillets)
- ½ cup white wine
- ½ cup non-fat yogurt mixed with ¼ cup pureed roasted red pepper
- ½ pound green beans
- ¾ pint cherry tomatoes (about 20)
- 1 tablespoon olive oil
- ¾ cup bulgur, prepared per package directions

Lightly dust fillets with flour. Dip in beaten egg white and then in Panko bread crumbs. Brown fillets in non-stick pan. Place fillets skin side down in baking dish coated with non-stick spray. Add white wine and cook in oven preheated to 350 °F for about 15 minutes. Spoon pan juices over fillets. Salt and pepper to taste.

Place green beans in skillet. Add ¼-inch of water and cook over medium heat until water boils off. Add cherry tomatoes and olive oil. Stir well and sauté for a few minutes. Season with fresh rosemary and oregano. Salt and pepper to taste.

Plate haddock fillet and spoon over yogurt-red pepper sauce. Garnish with fresh parsley. Add green beans & tomato mix and the bulgur.   Serve hot.

<u>Serves 4</u>. One plate consisting of one haddock fillet (215 Calories) with green beans & tomato mix (65 Calories) and bulgur (140 Calories) totals 420 Calories.

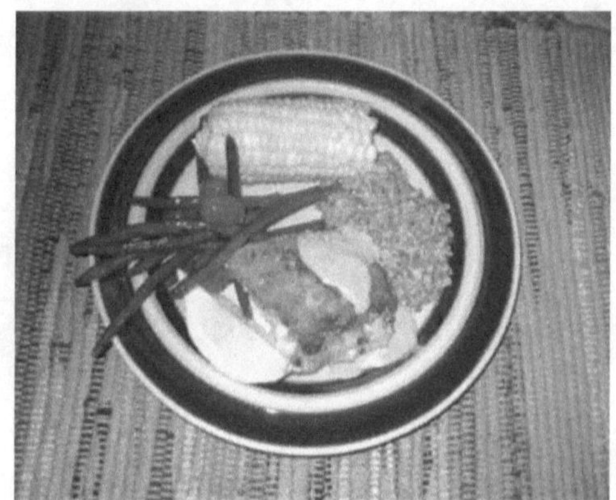

Note that corn-on-the-cob is only for the 1,800 Calorie diet.

<u>Diet Tip of the Day:</u> It's much easier to stay with an exercise program when it's done in tandem. So enlist a friend to be your exercise buddy.

<u>Chicken Cacciatore</u>

- ¾ lb skinless, boneless chicken breast halves
- ¼ lb of your favorite pasta
- ½ cup chopped onion
- ½ cup chopped green bell pepper
- 14.5-ounce can chopped tomatoes, drained
- 8-ounce can tomato sauce
- 1½ teaspoons Italian seasoning
- ⅓ cup sliced ripe olives
- ⅛ teaspoon black pepper

Cut chicken breasts into small pieces. Spray a large heavy skillet with olive oil flavored cooking spray.

Sauté chicken, onion and green pepper for 6 to 8 minutes. Stir in drained tomatoes and tomato sauce. Add Italian seasoning, olives and ⅛ teaspoon ground black pepper. Mix well to combine. Lower heat and simmer for 15 to 20 minutes, stirring occasionally.

Cook pasta per package directions. Ladle chicken and sauce over pasta and serve immediately.

<u>Serves 4</u>. About 310 Calories per serving

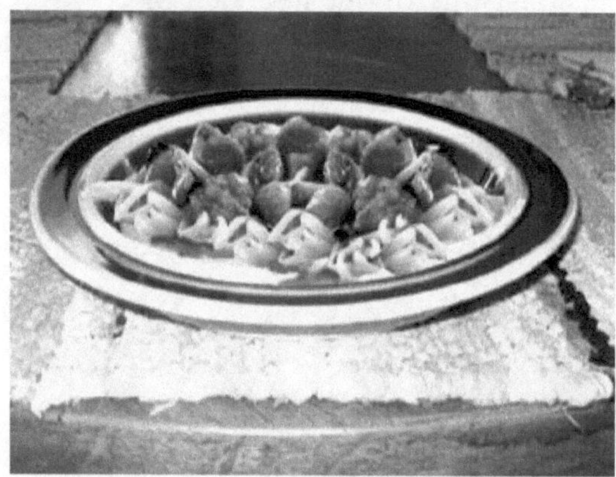

<u>Diet Tip of the Day</u>: Inevitably, you're going to be faced with a stressful situation. Instead of turning to food for comfort, be prepared with some non-food tactics that work for you, such as listening to music, reading, writing in a journal, or meditating.

Day 46 - Recipe

Poached Cod in Tomato Broth

    2   cups dry white wine
    1   cup clam juice
    2   cans (14.5-ounce) diced tomatoes, drained
    1   small onion, diced
    1   garlic clove, minced
    ½   tsp dried parsley, or sprigs of fresh parsley
    1   bay leaf
    12 black olives, pitted and halved
    4   cod fish fillets (about 6 ounces each)

Note that sole, flounder, halibut or haddock may be substituted for cod.

Use a pan large enough to hold the fish in a single layer. Place all the ingredients except the fish in the pan. Over high heat, bring poaching liquid to a boil (pan uncovered). Reduce heat and simmer the liquid another 6 minutes.

Carefully place the fish filets in the liquid. Cover the pan and reduce heat until liquid is just simmering. Poach until fish are completely opaque and tender – about 8 minutes. Plate fish and ladle broth over fish.
Serves 4. 275 Calories per serving.

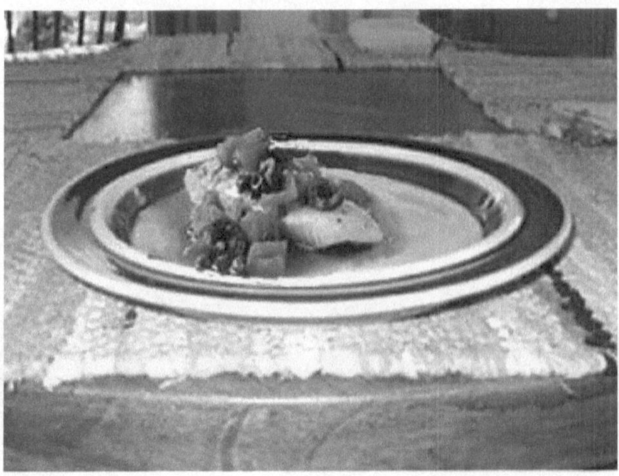

Diet Tip of the Day: **A good reducing diet must help you remain healthy** while you are losing weight.

Day 47 - Recipe

<u>Black-Eyed Peas over Rice</u>

  2 cups fat-free, lower-sodium chicken broth
  2 slices smoked bacon
  2 cups water
  ½ teaspoon kosher salt
  ½ teaspoon freshly ground black pepper
  1-pound bag frozen black-eyed peas, thawed
  12-ounce bunch fresh turnip greens, trimmed and coarsely chopped
  2 tablespoons pepper vinegar

Cook bacon in a Dutch oven over medium heat until crisp. Remove bacon from pan using a slotted spoon, reserving drippings in pan. Crumble bacon.

Add onion to drippings in pan; sauté 4 minutes, stirring occasionally. Stir in broth and the next 5 ingredients (through greens); bring to a boil. Reduce heat, and simmer for about an hour or until peas are tender, stirring occasionally and skimming as necessary. Stir in vinegar. Ladle about 1⅓ cups pea mixture into each of 4 bowls and top evenly with crumbled bacon. <u>Serves 4</u>. 280 Calories per serving (does not include rice)

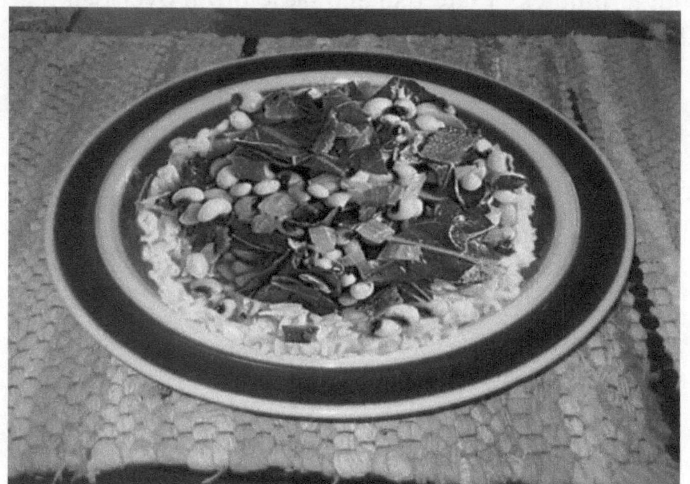

Two servings of black-eyed peas over brown rice on platter.

<u>Diet Tip of the Day:</u> Black-eyed peas are a wonderful food but **black-eyed peas are an incomplete protein**. If however black-eyed peas are eaten with a grain such as rice, the combination forms a complete protein – just as complete a protein as meat, poultry, or fish!

Day 48 - Recipe

<u>Healthy Pasta Salad</u>

½	pound fusilli pasta, cooked until tender but firm
2	broccoli crowns, chopped
¼	pint cherry tomatoes (about 8), halved
½	cup black olives, halved
½	cup garbanzo beans (chick peas)
½	cup fresh "light" mozzarella, chopped
1	tablespoon basil
1	tablespoon rosemary
2	teaspoons garlic powder
¼	cup of a recommended dressing on page 11.

Combine dry ingredients in a medium-size bowl. Stir in salad dressing. Mix thoroughly. Salt and black pepper to taste.

<u>Serves 4</u>. 370 Calories per serving.

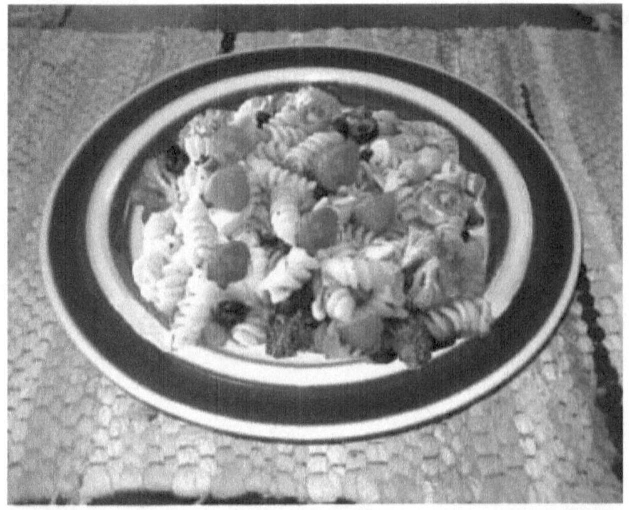

<u>**Diet Tip of the Day:**</u> Ask yourself: **"Why am I overweight**?" Do you eat too much of everything? Too much dessert? Drink too much beer? Is your only exercise walking from the TV to the refrigerator? Determine the why and then focus on one or two of your problem areas. Sometimes it's that simple.

Day 49 - Recipe

<u>Frozen-Meat Dinner</u>

No recipe today. No cooking today. It's your day off! To find a frozen meat dinner entrée please go to Appendix A (page 198) which lists approximately 150 frozen dinners manufactured by Healthy Choice, Lean Cuisine and Smart Ones.

Note that if you do not use all of the **300 Calories allocated for the Day 49 frozen dinner**, use the excess calories anyway you wish. Splurge on extra dessert or save the calories for another day.

Please read the important **Frozen-Food Safety Warning** in Appendix B on page 204.

<u>**Diet Tip of the Day:**</u> Experts agree that whether you are trying to lose weight or just maintain your weight, **it's calories that count**. It doesn't matter what foods the calories are from. To lose weight you must eat fewer calories than you burn. Calories count! Not carbs, not Weight Watchers points. Calories – period!

<h1 align="center">Day 50 - Recipe</h1>

<u>Pan-Fried Sole</u>

    4   sole fillets (6-ounces each), skinned
    1   tablespoon olive oil

<u>Salsa Ingredients</u>:
    1 pint cherry tomatoes, quartered
    ¾ cup cucumber, finely chopped
    ⅓ cup yellow bell pepper, finely chopped
    3 tablespoons fresh basil, chopped
    2 tablespoons capers
    1½ tablespoons shallots, finely chopped
    1 tablespoon balsamic vinegar
    2 teaspoons lemon rind, grated

Combine salsa ingredients in a bowl and stir in ½ teaspoon salt and ⅛ teaspoon black pepper. Mix thoroughly.

Heat olive oil in a large nonstick skillet over medium-high heat. Season sole fillets with
½ teaspoon salt and ⅛ teaspoon black pepper. Add fish to pan; cook about 1½ minutes on each side or until fish flakes easily when tested with a fork. Spoon salsa over fish and serve immediately.
<u>Serves 4</u>. 325 Calories per serving

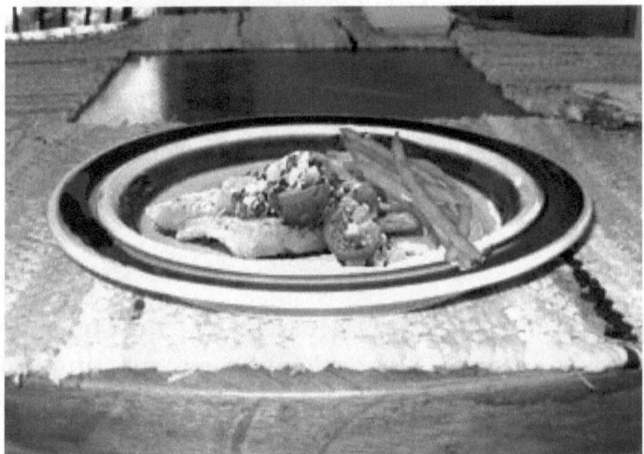

<u>Diet Tip of the Day:</u> If you are overweight start on a weight loss diet now because it will only become **more difficult to lose weight as you get older.**

Day 51 - Recipe

Beans & Greens Salad (Repeated)

⅓ cup chopped oregano
⅓ cup chopped parsley
3 cloves garlic, chopped
1 lemon, juiced

Prepare dressing by combining above ingredients and stirring in ¼ cup extra-virgin olive oil. Salt and pepper to taste.

½ pound mesclun mix
¼ pound green beans
19-ounce can garbanzo beans (chickpeas)

Arrange mesclun mix, garbanzo beans and green beans on a large platter. (Set aside one serving - about ¼ of the salad and ¼ of the dressing for lunch on Day 55. Combine left over dressing and salad when served.) Drizzle the remaining dressing over the rest of the salad.

<u>Serves 4</u>. Approximately 260 Calories per serving.

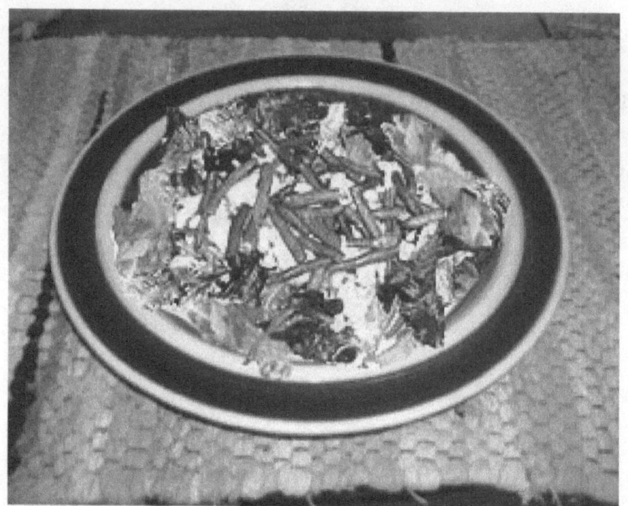

<u>**Diet Tip of the Day:**</u> **Fat-free isn't always your best bet**. Low fat doesn't necessarily mean low calorie! Most often sugar is substituted for fat and the calorie total remains the same or even higher. Instead, look for low-calorie or reduced-calorie foods.

<u>Chicken Piccata</u>

- 1 pound boneless skinless chicken breast halves
- 2 teaspoons olive oil
- 1 teaspoon minced garlic
- ¼ cup shallots, diced
- ¾ pound fresh green beans, washed and snipped
- 1 teaspoon lemon juice
- ¼ cup capers, rinsed
- 2 fresh lemons, cut into small wedges

In a skillet, heat olive oil and minced garlic over medium heat. Sauté chicken breasts and shallots for two to three minutes, tossing often, until chicken is partially cooked. Add green beans and one teaspoon of lemon juice and sauté for an additional two to three minutes, or until chicken is completely cooked and green beans are al dente. Add capers; and cover chicken. Let sit for one more minute to warm capers. Serve immediately with wedges of lemon.

<u>Serves 4</u>. 270 calories per serving

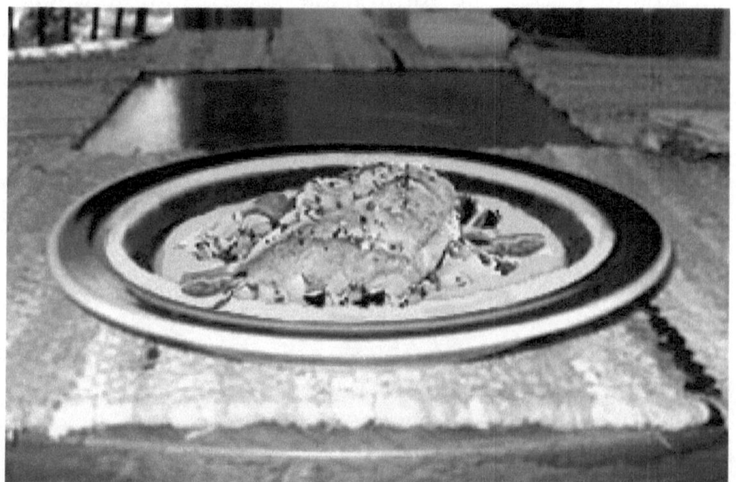

<u>Diet Tip of the Day:</u> Handle **occasional overeating by compensating**. To do this, estimate how far you have strayed from your weight-loss diet and then make amends at the next opportunity (usually the next meal or two) – by eating less.

Day 53 - Recipe

<u>Pasta Primavera</u>

 ½ pound fusilli whole-wheat pasta
 2 small yellow squash, halved and cut into ½-inch-thick slices
 1 medium orange bell pepper, cut into 1-inch pieces
 8 oz. small broccoli florets (3 cups)
 2 cups halved cherry tomatoes
 8 green onions, thinly sliced (½ cup)
 3 Tbs. olive oil
 3 cloves garlic, minced (about 1 Tbsp)
 ½ cup torn fresh basil leaves
 1 tsp. grated lemon zest

Combine oil, garlic, and lemon zest in small bowl. Set aside. Cook pasta in large pot of boiling, salted water according to package directions.   Add squash and bell pepper 4 minutes before end of cooking time. Add broccoli 3 minutes before end of cooking time. Drain pasta and vegetables, reserving ½ cup cooking water.

Return pasta mixture to pot, and stir in tomatoes, green onions, basil, oil mixture, and reserved cooking water. Heat over medium-low heat until tomatoes are hot. Serve with Parmesan cheese, if desired.
<u>Serves 4</u>. 350 Calories per serving

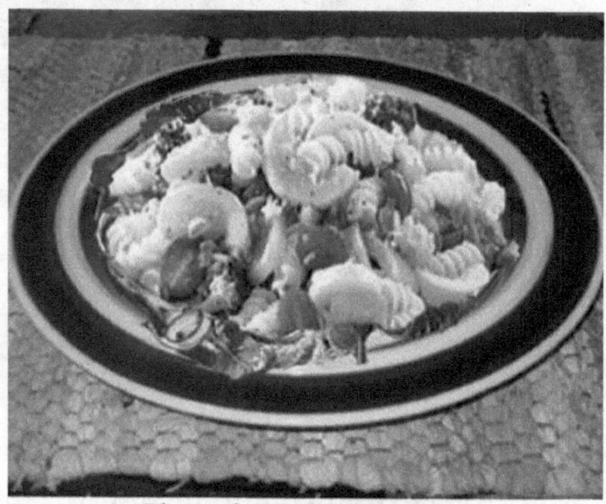

Photo shows two servings.

<u>Diet Tip of the Day:</u> **Beware of alcoholic beverages**. Beer has about 13 Calories per ounce, wine 25 Calories per ounce and whiskey a whopping 71 Calories per ounce.

Day 54 - Recipe

<u>Tina's Grilled Scallops &Polenta</u>

1 pound sea scallops
¾ cup polenta cornmeal
¾ cup skim milk
1 medium Portobello mushroom
½ pound green beans
¼ cup chopped red onion
16 asparagus spears
1 teaspoon extra-virgin olive oil

Bring 1½ cups of water and skim milk to rapid boil. Add salt to taste and slowly add polenta while stirring. Reduce heat. Continue stirring until desired consistency is reached. Pour polenta into lightly greased pan. After polenta has cooled cover and refrigerate. Cut chilled polenta into 4 pieces. Grill on medium-hot fire – about two minutes on each side.

Brush Portobello mushroom and asparagus spears with olive oil and place on grill for about 3 minutes on each side.

Grill scallops on medium-hot fire. Turn after two minutes or when first side turns opaque. Grill until second side turns opaque – about another 2 minutes. Don't overcook but test a scallop by cutting to make sure it's cooked through. Salt and pepper to taste.

<u>Serves 4</u>. The food on the plate pictured below totals about 380 Calories.

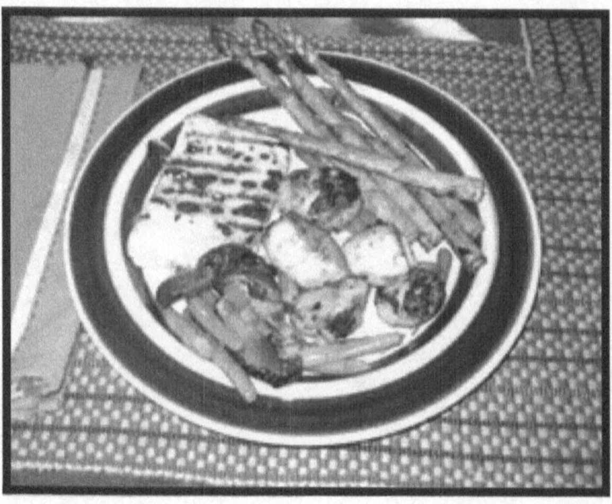

<u>Diet Tip of the Day:</u> To have better control of what you eat **bring your lunch to work**.

Day 55 - Recipe

Hearty Vegetable Soup

- 2 15-oz cans white kidney beans, drained
- 1 tablespoon olive oil
- ½ large yellow onion, chopped
- 2 garlic cloves, minced
- 1 cup chopped fresh tomatoes
- 2 celery stalks, cut into ½-inch pieces
- 1½ carrots, cut into ½-inch pieces
- 5 cups vegetable stock
- 1 medium potato, cut into ½-inch pieces
- ¼ cup chopped fresh basil
- ¼ head of red cabbage, cut into ½-inch pieces
- 2 zucchini or summer squash, cut into ½-inch pieces

Heat olive oil in a large pot over medium heat. Add onion and garlic. Sauté 5 minutes. Add green cabbage, tomatoes, celery, and carrots. Sauté 10 minutes. Add beans, 5 cups of stock, potatoes, and basil. Bring to a boil. Reduce heat, cover and simmer for one hour. Add red cabbage, zucchini and salt . Cover and simmer until vegetables are tender, about 20 minutes longer. Stir in about ¼ cup Parmesan cheese and sprinkle a dash of Tabasco hot sauce if you want a little zip

Serves 4. 360 Calories per serving

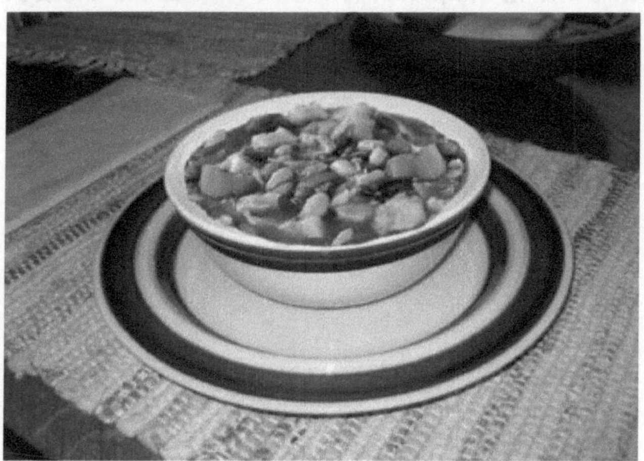

Diet Tip of the Day: Water and fiber contain no calories – that is **zero Calories** per ounce.

<h1 align="center">Day 56 - Recipe</h1>

<u>Frozen Chicken Dinner</u>

No recipe today. No cooking today. It's your day off! To find a frozen chicken dinner entrée please go to Appendix A (page 198) which lists approximately 150 frozen dinners manufactured by Healthy Choice, Lean Cuisine and Smart Ones.

Note that if you do not use all of the **300 Calories allocated for the Day 56 frozen dinner,** use the excess calories anyway you wish. Splurge on extra dessert or save the calories for another day.

Please read the important **Frozen-Food Safety Warning** in Appendix B on page 204.

<u>**Diet Tip of the Day**</u>: To prevent or delay the onset of type II diabetes, experts urge the overweight to lose weight and work out regularly. Weight loss helps your body use insulin more efficiently, and exercise helps metabolize excess circulating blood glucose.

Day 57 - Recipe

<u>Salmon with Mango Salsa</u>

  4 salmon fillets (about 5 ounces each)
  1½ pounds baby new potatoes, halved
  1 mango, ripe
  3 green onions, finely chopped
  3 tablespoons chopped fresh cilantro
  2 tablespoons lemon juice
  2 teaspoons extra-virgin olive oil
  4 cups watercress

Remove any tiny bones from salmon. Press crushed peppercorns into flesh side of salmon. Set aside. Place halved potatoes into saucepan. Cover with water and bring to a boil. Reduce the heat and simmer until tender, about 10-12 minutes and drain.

Prepare salsa: Peel and seed the mango. Dice the mango flesh and put into a large bowl. Mix in green onions, cilantro, lemon juice, olive oil, and an optional dash of Tabasco.

Heat a grill pan coated with nonstick cooking spray over medium-high heat. Place salmon fillets in pan, skin-side down. Cook for 4 minutes. Turn fish over and cook until done, about another 4 minutes. Arrange watercress and new potatoes on serving plates. Place salmon on top and spoon over mango salsa.

<u>Serves 4</u>. 460 Calories per serving

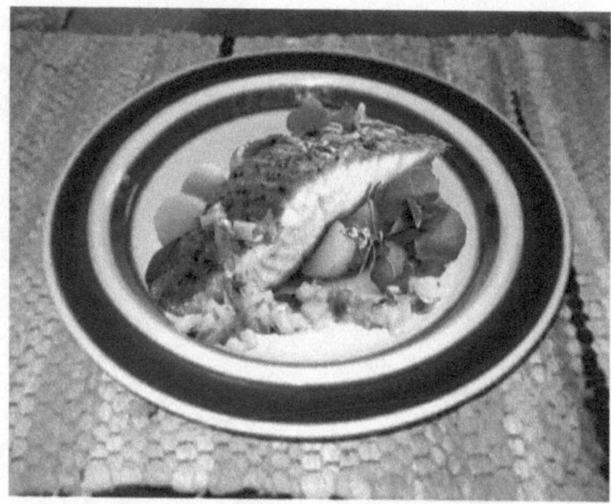

<u>Diet Tip of the Day:</u> All **foods are a combination of water, carbohydrate, protein, fat and fiber**. Knowing this can lead to a better understanding of why a food has a particular caloric value.

Pork Chop with Orange Slices

4	loin pork chops, ½-inch-thick (about 1½ lbs total, including bones)
8	orange slices, ¼-inch-thick
1	teaspoon salt
¾	teaspoon black pepper
¼	cup orange marmalade preserve
½	cup bottled fruit-based barbecue sauce

such as Grandville's Gourmet BBQ Sauce

<u>Marinade</u>: ½ cup orange juice, 2 teaspoons soy sauce and ¼ teaspoon crushed red pepper.

Combine pork chops and marinade in large re-sealable plastic bag. Refrigerate for about 30 minutes. Remove chops from marinade and season with salt and black pepper.

Stir together orange marmalade and BBQ sauce in a small bowl. Brush one side of pork chops evenly with half of marmalade-BBQ mixture. Grill chops, with marmalade-BBQ mixture side up over medium-high heat (about 375°) for about 5 minutes or until done. Turn chops, and brush with remaining marmalade-BBQ mixture. Grill another 5 minutes or until done. Grill orange slices over medium-high heat, 1 minute on each side.

<u>Serves 4</u>. 470 Calories per serving (includes pork chop and two orange slices).

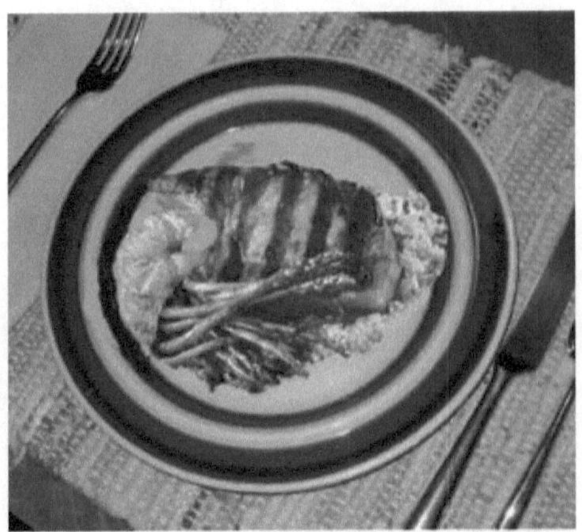

<u>Diet Tip of the Day:</u> Make sure fat is trimmed from meat. Most meats are about 80 Calories per ounce – whereas, pure fat is 256 Calories per ounce!

Day 59 - Recipe

<u>Fish Dinner - Out</u>

No recipe today. No cooking today. Have a fish dinner at your favorite restaurant, but make sure you choose a restaurant where you have a good chance to achieve your calorie goal. For today, your **goal for dinner is a maximum of 595 Calories**. This includes appetizer, soup, main course and dessert.

Tips for Eating Fish Out: The following is almost an exact repeat of the advice given eating out on previous days. First order simple, such as broiled fish with steamed vegetables and brown rice. Tell the waiter you want no sauce, no gravy, nothing added. Then, knowing your calorie objective, and that fish is about 50 Calories per ounce, most steamed vegetable servings average approximately 50 Calories per cup, and rice is about 100 Calories per ½ cup, decide how much to eat – and take the remainder home. If fresh fruit is not an option, pass on dessert and have the evening snack specified for that day in the diet.

In a restaurant, some nutritionists recommend you eat the low-calorie items on your plate first. Start with the salad, soup and veggies. By the time you get to the fish and starches you will hopefully be full enough to be content with smaller portions of the higher-calorie choices.

<u>Diet Tip of the Day:</u> A handful of studies suggest that chewing gum may help reduce your craving for sweet snacks, and cut your caloric intake by about 50 per day. Another study actually showed that gum chewers experienced a small increase in their daily energy expenditure. And gum adds hardly any calories to your diet. Regular gum has about 10 calories and sugar-free varieties about five calories per stick.

Day 60 - Recipe

<u>Chicken Stew over Rice</u>

4	boneless skinless chicken breasts (about 1 lb)
1	medium Onion
3	stalks celery
12	mushrooms
2	cups baby carrots
3	cups broccoli florets
½	teaspoon black pepper
¼	teaspoon herb seasoning blend
2	teaspoons Worcestershire Sauce
1	bay leaf
1	cup Cream of Chicken Soup (Campbell's)

Prepare a large, heavy, stove-top pot with cooking spray. Sauté at medium-high heat finely chop onion until caramelized. Cut chicken into bite size pieces and add to pot. Cook and toss until chicken is no longer pink. Add black pepper, herb seasoning and Worcestershire sauce. Stir. Add sliced celery and mushrooms, and then broccoli, carrots and bay leaf. Pour in Cream of Chicken soup. Gradually add one cup water while stirring. (You may want to add more water to get consistency desired.) Simmer until hot and flavors have combined. Serve over rice.

<u>Serves 4.</u> 360 Calories per serving (not including the brown rice below the stew).

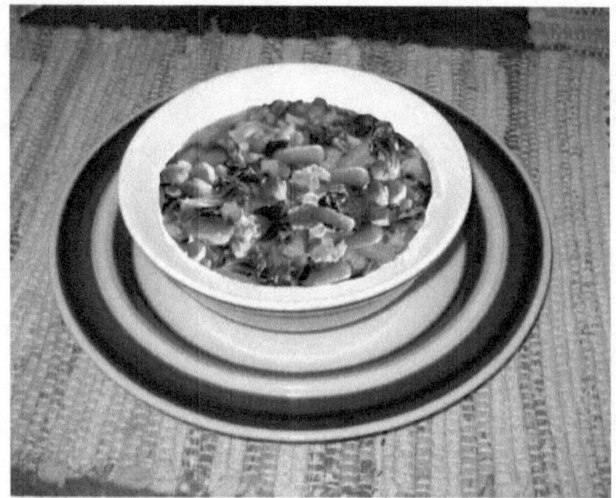

<u>Diet Tip of the Day:</u> Studies show people who eat 5 to 6 **mini-meals** and snacks a day don't feel as hungry and are better able to control their appetite and their weight.

Day 61 - Recipe

<u>Shrimp over Spaghetti</u>

- ½ lb spaghetti
- 1 lb shrimp, peeled and de-veined
- 6 ounces dry white wine
- 3 tablespoons olive oil
- 3 cloves garlic, sliced thin
- ¼ cup chopped basil leaves

Cook spaghetti according to package directions. Save ½ cup of the pasta cooking water.

In a large skillet over medium heat, cook olive oil and garlic, stirring until garlic turns golden, and then discard garlic. Add shrimp and increase heat to medium-high and stir in chopped basil leaves, white wine and ½ cup cooking water. Cook another 2 to 3 minutes or until shrimp are just firm. Spoon shrimp and sauce over spaghetti. Season with salt and black pepper. Garnish with parsley.

<u>Serves 4</u>. 450 Calories per serving

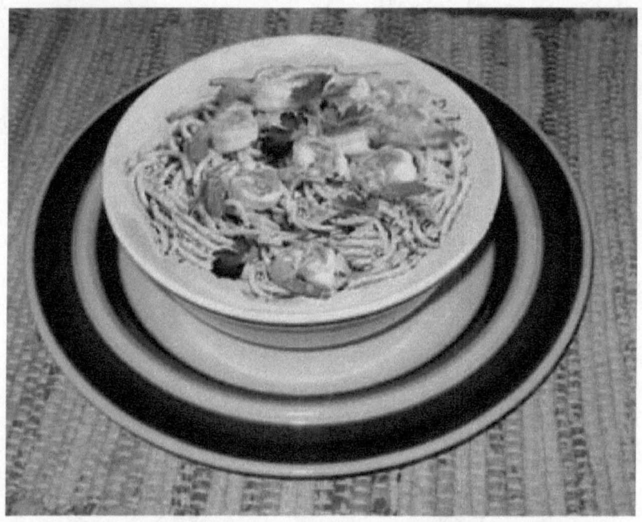

<u>Diet Tip of the Day:</u> If your caloric intake on a weight-loss diet is constant, your **rate of weight loss will decrease with time**. So if you want to lose weight at a constant rate over time, you must eat slightly less (or exercise harder) as you lose weight.

Day 62 - Recipe

<u>Beef Burgundy</u>

- 1 lb boneless beef chuck, trimmed & cut in 1" pieces
- 2 large carrots, cut into 1-inch pieces
- 1 medium onion, cut into 1-inch pieces
- 1 tablespoon flour
- 1 tablespoon tomato paste
- 1 clove garlic, crushed
- 1 tablespoon olive oil
- 1 cup dry red wine
- 2 sprigs fresh thyme
- 10 ounces mushrooms, sliced in half
- 8 ounces frozen peas

In Dutch oven, heat oil on medium-high until hot. Add beef and cook 5 to 6 minutes or until beef is browned on all sides. Transfer beef to a bowl. Preheat oven to 325° F. To drippings in Dutch oven, add carrots, garlic, and onion. Stir occasionally and cook 10 minutes or until vegetables are browned and tender. Stir in flour, tomato paste, ½ teaspoon salt, and ¼ teaspoon black pepper, and cook another minute. Add wine and heat to boiling, stirring until browned bits are loosened from bottom of Dutch oven. Return meat and any juices in the bowl to Dutch oven. Add thyme and mushrooms; bring to a boil. Cover and bake 1½ hours or until meat is fork-tender. Discard thyme sprigs. Before stew is done, cook peas per package instructions and add peas to Dutch oven.

<u>Serves 4</u>. 350 Calories per serving

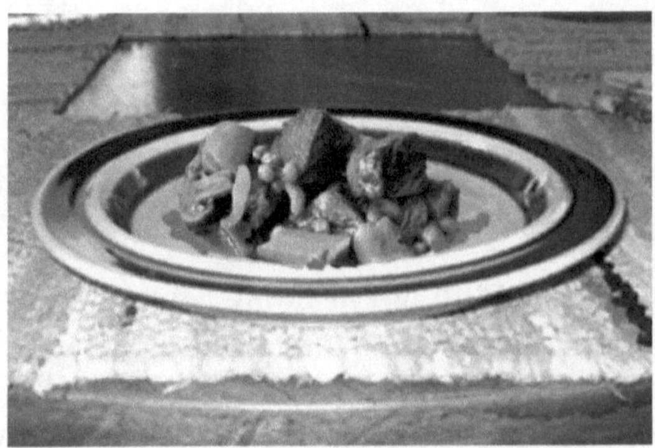

<u>Diet Tip of the Day:</u> When on a diet **simple is better**. Why? Because simple, uncomplicated meals usually contain fewer "hidden calories" than more elaborate dishes.

Day 63 - Recipe

<u>Chicken Cutlet</u>

Buy 4 skinless, boneless chicken cutlets or breast halves (about 1 lb), flattened to about ¼ to ½-inch thick.

   ¾ cup Panko bread crumbs
   ⅓ cup grated Parmesan cheese
   1   egg, beaten
   4   tablespoons extra-virgin olive oil, divided

Season chicken cutlets with salt and pepper. Combine bread crumbs and Parmesan cheese in a shallow bowl. Whisk egg in a separate shallow bowl. Dip chicken in egg and then coat both sides in crumb mixture.

Heat 2 tablespoons of olive oil in large skillet over medium-high heat. Add 2 cutlets, and cook 2 minutes on each side or until cooked through. Repeat with 2 tablespoons olive oil and remaining 2 cutlets. Serve hot.
<u>Serves 4.</u> 450 Calories per serving (chicken cutlet only)

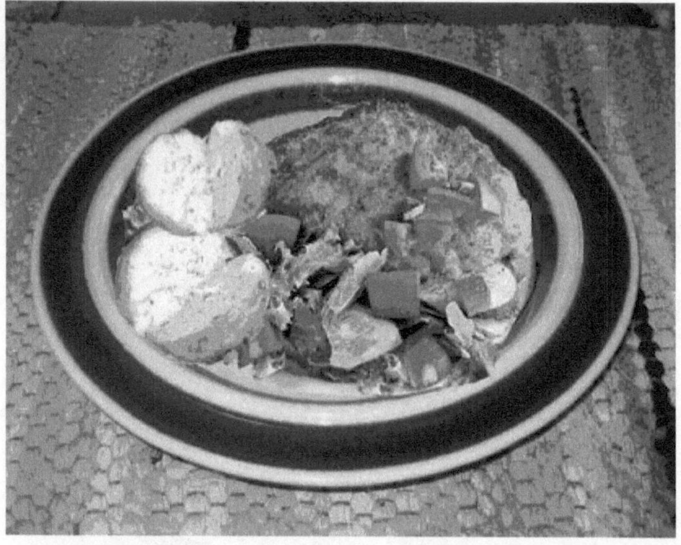

<u>Diet Tip of the Day:</u> **Working out at home** has some significant advantages. Your workout takes less time because you don't have to drive back and forth to a fitness facility; and you have the flexibility of dividing your workout into small time segments to fit your day, and working out at home is less expensive.

<u>Turkey Meat Loaf</u>

- 1½ cups finely chopped onion
- 1 tablespoon minced garlic
- 1 teaspoon olive oil
- 1 medium carrot, cut into ¼-inch pieces
- ¾ pound cremini mushrooms, finely chopped
- 1 teaspoon salt & ½ teaspoon black pepper
- 1½ teaspoons Worcestershire sauce
- ⅓ cup fresh parsley, finely chopped
- ¼ cup plus 1 tablespoon ketchup
- 1 cup fresh bread crumbs
- ⅓ cup 1% milk
- 1 whole large egg, & large egg white, lightly beaten
- 1¼ pound ground turkey (mostly light meat)

Preheat oven to 400°F. Cook onion and garlic in oil in a 12-inch nonstick skillet over moderate heat, stirring, until onion is softened, about 2 minutes. Add carrot and cook, stirring, until softened, about 3 minutes. Add mushrooms, ½ teaspoon salt, and ¼ teaspoon pepper and cook, stirring occasionally, until mushrooms are very tender, 10 to 15 minutes. Stir in Worcestershire sauce, parsley, and 3 tablespoons ketchup. Transfer vegetable mixture to a large bowl and cool.

Stir together bread crumbs and milk in a small bowl and let stand 5 minutes. Stir in egg and egg white, then add to vegetable mixture. Add turkey and remaining ½ teaspoon salt and ¼ teaspoon pepper to vegetable mixture and mix well. (Mixture will be very moist.)

Form into a 9 x 5-inch oval loaf in a lightly oiled 13 x 9 x 2-inch metal baking pan and brush meat loaf evenly with remaining 2 tablespoons ketchup. Bake in middle of oven until thermometer inserted into meat loaf registers 170°F, about 50 to 55 minutes. Let meat loaf stand 5 minutes. **<u>Serves 6</u>**. 240 Calories per serving

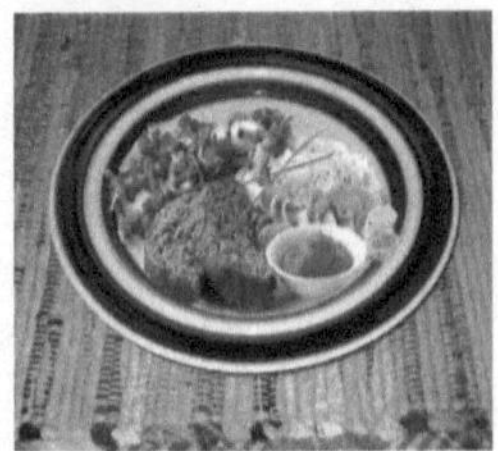

Photo shows meat loaf with noodles & mixed greens.

Day 65 - Recipe

Frozen-Fish Dinner

No recipe today. No cooking today. It's your day off! To find a frozen fish dinner, please go to Appendix A (page 198) which lists approximately 150 frozen dinners manufactured by Healthy Choice, Lean Cuisine and Smart Ones.

Perusing the list, it is obvious that there are not many frozen fish dinners for sale at supermarkets. Note that if you do not use all of the **340 Calories allocated for this Day 5 meal**, use the excess calories anyway you wish. Splurge on extra dessert or save the calories for the next day and have a larger piece of pizza!

Please read the important **Frozen-Food Safety Warning** in Appendix B on page 204.

Diet Tip of the Day: **Muscle** is active tissue, fat is not. The more muscle you have, the more calories you burn. Muscle uses a significant number of calories every day for repair and rebuilding, giving your metabolism a boost even when you're resting. So make sure strengthening exercises (like weight lifting) are part of your workout.

<u>Pita Pizza</u>

> 6 pita bread loaves (Joseph's Flax, Oat Bran & Whole Wheat Pita Bread -
> 8 oz pkg)
> ¾ cup part-skim shredded mozzarella, divided
> 1 large red pepper, sliced
> 1 medium onion, sliced
> 6 medium mushrooms, sliced
> ¾ cup tomato sauce, divided
> 4 tablespoons olive oil

Cook olive oil in large skillet over medium-high heat. Add pepper slices, onion slices and mushroom slices and sauté until they softened.

Toast pita loaves slightly (so they don't get soggy when sauce is applied). Coat one side of pita with tomato sauce. Arrange pepper, onion and mushroom slices on individual pita loaves and sprinkle shredded mozzarella cheese on top.

In oven preheated to 400°F, place pita loaves on baking tin coated with cooking spray. Cook approximately 5 minutes or until cheese melts. Season with salt and pepper to taste.

<u>Serves 3</u>. 430 Calories per serving (Two Pita Pizzas per serving.)

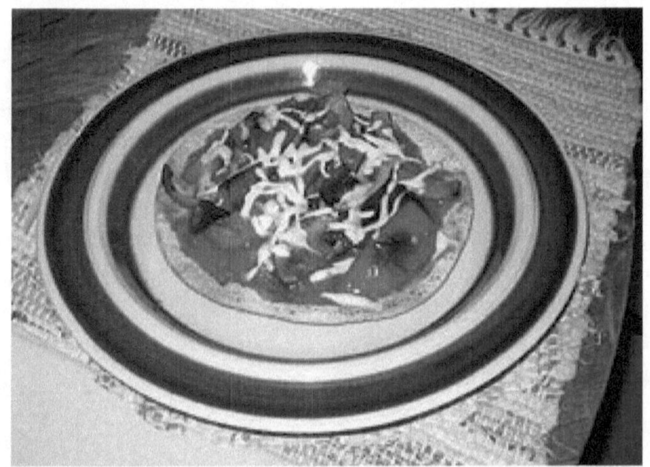

Note only one pita pizza shown. Serving size is <u>two</u> pita pizzas.

<u>**Diet Tip of the Day:**</u> On a reducing diet, **when you lose – you win**! You win a much better chance for a longer healthier life, you win a sense of well-being, you win a more attractive appearance – and finally you win a feeling of accomplishment.

Day 67 - Recipe

<u>Chicken Dinner - Out</u>

No recipe today. No cooking today. Have a chicken dinner at your favorite restaurant, but make sure you choose a restaurant where you have a fighting chance to achieve your calorie goal. For your chicken dinner out, your maximum allowable calories (includes appetizer, soup, main course and dessert) are as follows:
   - For **1,200 Calorie Diet**: 530 Calories
   - For **1,500 Calorie Diet**: 630 Calories

Tips for Eating Chicken Out: First, order simple and order skinless white meat only, such as broiled chicken breast with steamed vegetables and brown rice. Tell the waiter you want no sauce, no gravy, nothing added. Then, knowing your calorie objective, and that chicken is about 50 Calories per ounce, most steamed vegetable servings average approximately 50 Calories per cup, and rice is about 100 Calories per ½ cup, decide how much to eat – and take the remainder home. If fresh fruit is not an option, pass on dessert and have the evening snack specified for that day in this diet.

In a restaurant, some nutritionists recommend you eat the low-calorie items on your plate first. Start with the salad, soup and veggies. By the time you get to the chicken and starches you will hopefully be full enough to be content with smaller portions of the higher-calorie choices. (Incidentally, feel free to substitute skinless white meat turkey for chicken.)

Finally, some dieticians advise their dieting clients not to eat out. That's right. They believe eating at home is safer. But our thought is you have to eat out eventually so why not learn how while your resolve is high?

<u>Diet Tip of the Day</u>: When you're eating out, consider **ordering children's portions** or a small sandwich as a way to trim calories and get the size of your meals under control.

<h1 style="text-align:center">Day 68 - Recipe</h1>

<u>Pork Medallions in Lime Sauce</u>

1   pound pork tenderloin
⅓   cup all purpose flour
2   tablespoons olive oil
1   tablespoon unsalted butter
½   cup of white wine
¼   cup lime juice
2   stalks celery, chopped
1   medium onion, chopped

Trim away the thin silver skin on the tenderloin and all visible fat. Discard trimmings. Cut tenderloin into ½ to ¾ inch thick medallions. Sprinkle medallions with salt and pepper. Place flour in a shallow dish and coat pork medallions. Warm olive oil in a large skillet over medium-low heat. Working in batches if necessary, cook pork medallions, turning once, until well browned on both sides, about 5 minutes total. (Note internal pork temperature should be 160º F.) Transfer pork to a plate.

Add the wine and lime juice to skillet and bring to boil, scraping up browned bits from bottom of pan with wooden spoon and stirring occasionally, until thickened, about 4 minutes. Remove from heat; stir in butter, chopped celery and onion. Return pork to pan and warm though, turning medallions to coat with sauce.

<u>Serves 4</u>. 450 Calories per serving (pork medallions and sauce only)

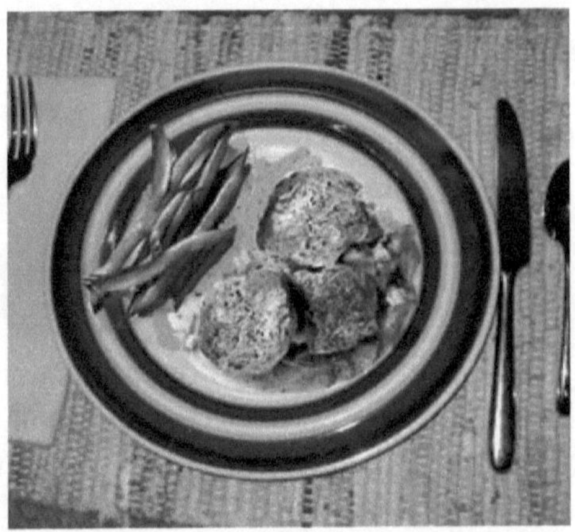

<u>Diet Tip of the Day:</u> Protein and carbohydrates are about 4 Calories per gram (110 Calories per ounce) and fat is 9 Calories per gram (260 Calories per ounce).

175

Day 69 - Recipe

Healthy Chicken Salad

4	skinless, boneless chicken breast halves, cooked
2	beefsteak tomatoes, cut into large pieces
1	celery heart, chopped
¼	pound roasted red peppers, from jar, chopped
1	small red onion, peeled, halved
10	black olives, halved
1	small bunch basil, leaves only
1½	tablespoons red wine vinegar
3	tablespoons extra-virgin olive oil
¼	pound croutons

Shred cooked chicken and mix with croutons, tomatoes, celery, roasted peppers, red onion, olives and basil in large bowl and season with salt and black pepper. Drizzle with 3 tablespoons extra-virgin olive oil and balsamic vinegar and toss.

Serves 4. 330 Calories per serving

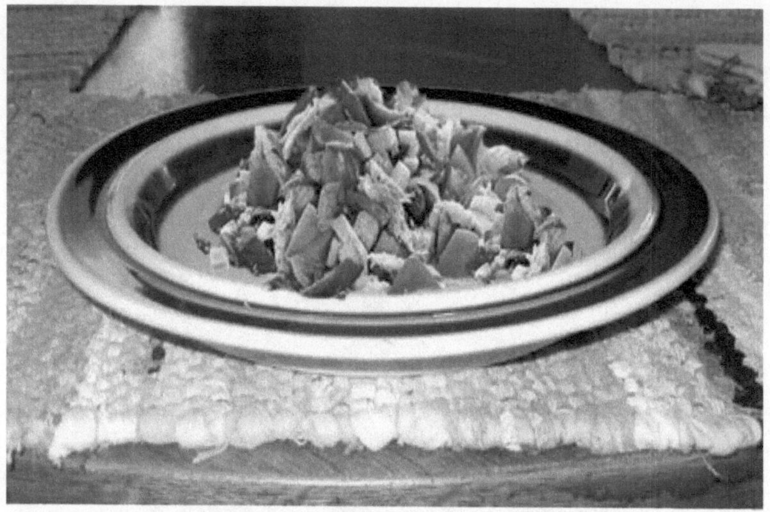

Diet Tip of the Day: In the view of many nutritionists, if you can afford it, buy local and **organic** but you don't have to buy organic across the board because not all organic-labeled products offer added health value.

<u>Baked Cod</u>

    4 cod fish fillets (4 to 5 ounces each)
    2 tablespoons flour
    2 tablespoons cornmeal
    2 tablespoons minced fresh herbs
    2 teaspoons lemon juice

Sprinkle cod with lemon juice. Mix flour, cornmeal and herbs and dust the cod with the cornmeal-herb mixture. Bake in oven at 375 °F for 10 minutes. Add salt and black pepper to taste.

<u>Serves 4</u>. One serving is 230 Calories (cod only).

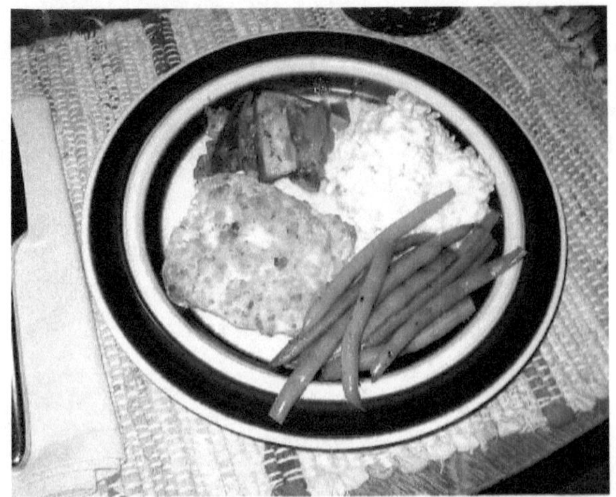

<u>Diet Tip of the Day:</u> It's worth **buying organic** for the "dirty dozen": peaches, strawberries, nectarines, apples, spinach, celery, pears, sweet bell peppers, cherries, potatoes, lettuce, and imported grapes. These fragile fruits and vegetables often require more pesticides to fight off bugs.

<u>Chicken Scaloppini</u>

- 4 skinless, boneless 6-oz chicken breast halves
- 2 teaspoons fresh lemon juice
- ⅓ cup Italian-seasoned breadcrumbs
- ½ cup fat-free, less-sodium chicken broth
- ¼ cup dry white wine
- 4 teaspoons capers
- 1 tablespoon extra-virgin olive oil

Place each chicken breast half between 2 sheets heavy-duty plastic wrap and pound to about ¼-inch thick using meat mallet. Cut each breast in quarters. Brush chicken with juice, and sprinkle with salt and black pepper. Dredge chicken in breadcrumbs.

Heat a large nonstick skillet coated with cooking spray over medium-high heat. Add chicken to pan; cook 3 minutes on each side or until chicken is done. Remove from pan; keep warm.

Add broth and wine to pan, and cook 30 seconds, stirring constantly. Remove from heat. Stir in capers and olive oil – and serve immediately. <u>Serves 4</u>. 260 Calories per serving (chicken only)

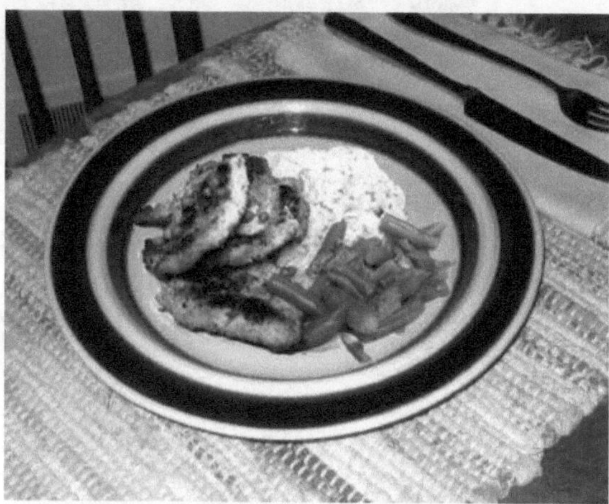

Chicken slightly burned, but still delicious!

<u>**Diet Tip of the Day**</u>: Nutritionists define a **"junk food"** as a food that offers little if any essential nutrients – except calories – and when eaten it replaces more important foods.

<u>Fish Dinner - Out</u>

No recipe today. No cooking today. Have a fish dinner at your favorite restaurant, but make sure you choose a restaurant where you have a good chance to achieve your calorie goal. For today, your **goal for dinner is a maximum of 595 Calories**. This includes appetizer, soup, main course, dessert and wine.

Tips for Eating Fish Out: The following is almost an exact repeat of the advice given eating out on previous days. First, order simple, such as broiled fish with steamed vegetables and brown rice. Tell the waiter you want no sauce, no gravy, nothing added. Then, knowing your calorie objective, and that fish is about 50 Calories per ounce, most steamed vegetable servings average approximately 50 Calories per cup, and rice is about 100 Calories per ½ cup, decide how much to eat – and take the remainder home. If fresh fruit is not an option, pass on dessert and have the evening snack specified for that day in the diet.

In a restaurant, some nutritionists recommend you eat the low-calorie items on your plate first. Start with the salad, soup and veggies. By the time you get to the fish and starches you will hopefully be full enough to be content with smaller portions of the higher-calorie choices.

<u>Diet Tip of the Day:</u> In the U.S., we consume more than 100 pounds of **sugar** per year per person, totaling an unhealthy, nutritionally empty, 500 Calories per day. This large intake of sugar leads to obvious ills, such as obesity and tooth decay.

Day 73 - Recipe

<u>Pasta Pomodoro</u>

Pasta Pomodoro (Italian for pasta with tomatoes) is typically prepared with angel hair pasta, olive oil, fresh tomatoes, and fresh basil. It's light, delicious and easy to make.

¾	pound angel hair pasta
1½	pints cherry tomatoes (about 45), halved
8	fresh basil leaves, chopped
4	cloves garlic, minced
2	tablespoons olive oil
4	Tbsp grated parmesan cheese

Cook angel hair pasta per package directions. Over medium heat, sauté the garlic in olive oil until it just starts to turn golden. Add tomatoes and cook for about 10 minutes, or until they just start to release juices. Turn off the heat and stir basil into the sauce. Over the cooked pasta, spoon the tomato sauce with a little of the pasta water and garnish with more basil and grated cheese.

<u>Serves 4</u>. 420 Calories per serving

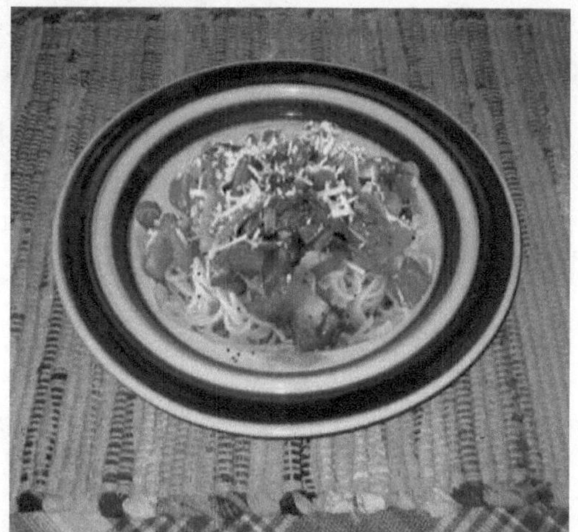

Above prepared with mix of cherry and plum tomatoes.

<u>Diet Tip of the Day:</u> Thinking about using **honey** rather than sugar? Honey has about 21 calories per teaspoon while sugar has 15. And the vitamin and mineral content of honey is very low.

Day 74 - Recipe

Frozen Chicken Dinner

No recipe today. No cooking today. It's your day off! To find a frozen chicken dinner entrée please go to Appendix A (page 198) which lists approximately 150 frozen dinners manufactured by Healthy Choice, Lean Cuisine and Smart Ones.

Note that if you do not use all of the **300 Calories allocated for the Day 56 frozen dinner**, use the excess calories anyway you wish. Splurge on extra dessert or save the calories for another day.

Please read the important **Frozen-Food Safety Warning** in Appendix B on page 204.

<u>**Diet Tip of the Day:**</u> Many health care professionals think that eating a healthy **vegetarian diet** is one of the best things you can do for your short-term and long-term health. But a vegetarian diet must be carefully planned.

Day 75 - Recipe

<u>Mediterranean Chicken</u>

4 small boneless skinless chicken breasts (about 1 lb total)
1 tablespoon paprika
1 tablespoon olive oil
½ teaspoon snipped fresh rosemary
2 cloves garlic, minced
¼ teaspoon ground black pepper
¼ cup dry red wine
3 tablespoons balsamic vinegar

Place chicken breast halves between two pieces of plastic wrap and pound with the flat side of a meat mallet into a rectangle ¼ to ½ inch thick. In a small bowl, combine paprika, oil, rosemary, garlic, and pepper; mixing well until it becomes a paste. Rub both sides of each chicken breast with paste mixture. Coat a 13x9x2-inch baking pan with nonstick cooking spray. Place coated chicken in prepared pan; cover and refrigerate for 2 to 6 hours.

Preheat oven to 450ºF. Drizzle chicken with wine. Bake for 6 to 8 minutes or until the chicken is no longer pink and a meat thermometer inserted in the thickest portion of the chicken registers 170ºF and the juices run clear. Turn the chicken once halfway through baking.

Remove from oven. Immediately drizzle vinegar onto chicken in the baking pan. Transfer chicken to serving plates. Stir the liquid in the baking pan and drizzle over chicken. If desired, garnish with fresh rosemary.
<u>Serves 4</u>. 180 Calories per serving (not including spaghetti squash & green beans)

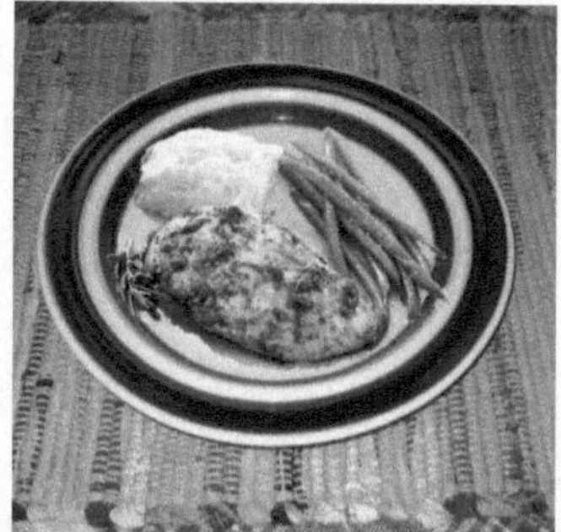

Photo shows chicken with spaghetti squash & green beans.

<u>Diet Tip of the Day:</u> Hunger is your body's way of telling you that you need calories. But **when you're done eating, you should feel better – satisfied but not stuffed**.

Day 76 - Recipe

<u>Gary & Sue's Grilled Scallops</u>

We were invited by our good friends, Gary and Sue, for dinner. They prepared a simple, but nutritious low-calorie meal – which featured scallops. (Scallops are a very low calorie food – expensive but great when you're on a diet.) The photo below is our version of the main course they served that night.

1½	pounds sea scallops
3	medium tomatoes, sliced, divided
4	ears of corn
2	tablespoons olive oil, divided
1	tablespoon balsamic vinegar, divided

Place scallops in a shallow bowl. Add olive oil and vinegar and toss to coat. Grill scallops on medium-hot fire. Turn after two minutes or when first side turns opaque. Grill until second side turns opaque – about another 2 minutes. Don't overcook but test a scallop by cutting to make sure it's cooked through. Salt and black pepper to taste.

<u>Serves 4</u>. The food pictured on the plate below totals about 360 Calories.

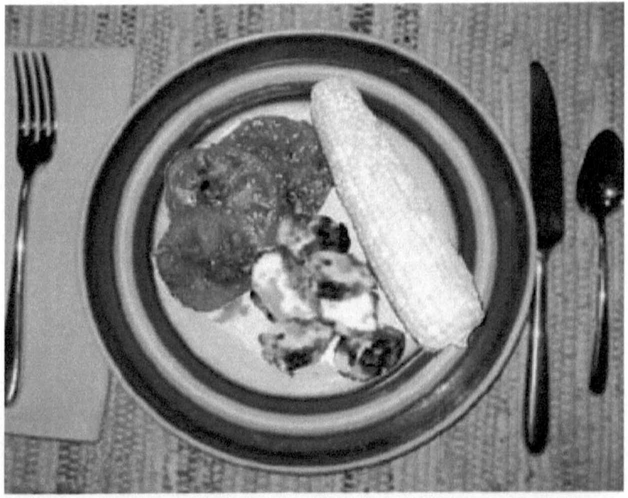

<u>**Diet Tip of the Day:**</u> When you eat fiber, it simply passes straight through, untouched by but aiding your digestive system. **Zero calories absorbed!**

Day 77 - Recipe

<u>Chicken with Peppers and Rice</u>

4   boneless, skinless chicken breast halves (about 1 lb)
1   red bell pepper, sliced
1   green bell pepper, sliced
1   yellow bell pepper, sliced
1   medium onion, sliced
1   ounce package of herb, garlic dip and soup mix
2   tablespoons olive oil
¾   cup wild rice, brown rice and wheat-berry mix.

Prepare wild rice per package directions. Cut chicken into 2 to 3-inch pieces.
Place vegetables and chicken in re-sealable plastic bag. Add seasoning blend
and olive oil. Seal bag and refrigerate for about two hours.

Preheat oven to 400°F. Place chicken and peppers in foil-lined baking pan.
(Discard any remaining liquid in bag.) Bake 30 to 40 minutes, or until
chicken is done. Broil an additional 2 to 3 minutes to brown chicken
(optional).

<u>Serves 4</u>. 290 Calories per serving (Chicken, peppers and wild rice)

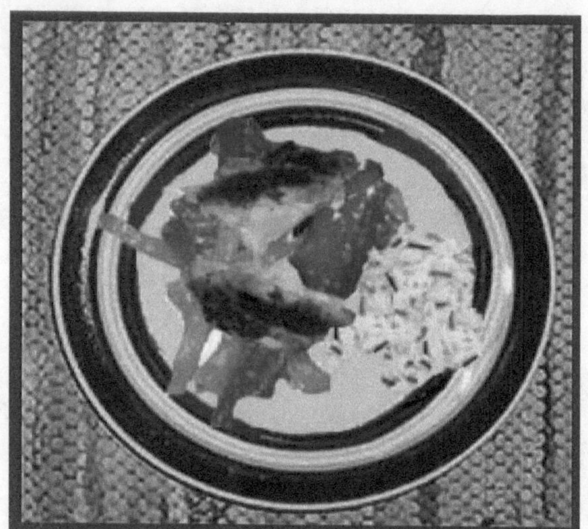

Chicken was browned too much but was still quite tasty!

<u>Diet Tip of the Day:</u> Most Americans consume too much sodium (salt).
The U.S. Department of Agriculture Dietary Guidelines recommend that
healthy adults **limit sodium intake to 2,400 mg per day**. (One teaspoon of
salt contains about 2,300 mg of sodium.)

<u>Trout with Lemon & Capers</u>

  4   trout fillets (4-oz each), skin attached
  3   tablespoons unsalted butter, divided
  2   tablespoons olive oil
  2   tablespoons lemon juice
  4   teaspoons chopped parsley
  1   teaspoon capers
  2   small lemons peeled and segmented

Score 2 crosswise slits (skin deep only) into each trout fillet using sharp knife. Turn the fillets over and season flesh with the salt and pepper.

Heat 1 tablespoon butter and the olive oil in a large nonstick skillet over medium-high heat. Place the fillets in the nonstick skillet, skin side up, and cook until golden brown, about 3 minutes. Turn and continue until cooked through and the skin begins to crisp around edges, about 2 more minutes. Transfer fillets to serving dish and keep warm.

Add the remaining 2 tablespoons butter to the hot skillet and cook until just brown. Stir in the lemon juice, parsley, capers, and lemon segments. Pour sauce over fillets and serve.

<u>Serves 4</u>. 340 Calories per serving (trout and sauce only)

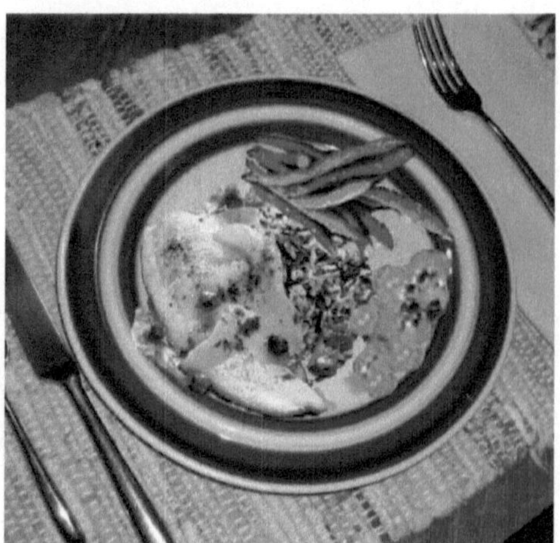

<u>Diet Tip of the Day:</u> Nearly every animal food, including dairy products, eggs, meat, poultry and fish are **complete proteins** because they contain all eight-essential amino acids. Soy is the only plant-based food that has all eight essential-amino acids.

Day 79 - Recipe

Italian Food - Out

No recipe today. No cooking today. Have dinner at your favorite Italian restaurant, but make sure you choose a restaurant where you have a reasonable chance to achieve your calorie goal. For today, **your goal for dinner is a maximum of 640 Calories**. This includes any appetizer, soup, main course and a 4 ounce glass of wine.

Tips for Eating Italian: You can consume a lot of calories in an Italian restaurant – if you order carelessly. For example a typical portion is often loaded with about 1000 Calories, then add another 100 Calories for a glass of wine.

First rule, order simple. Look for a dish with lots of vegetables, some fish or chicken. Then, knowing your 640 Calorie objective, and that chicken and fish are about 50 Calories per ounce, most steamed vegetable servings average approximately 50 Calories per cup, and pasta is about 200 Calories per cup, decide how much of the meal you can eat – and take the remainder the diet. Also see Eating Out (page 11) for more guidance.

Incidentally, although Italian is specified, feel free to substitute any other favorite ethnic food. Just make sure you don't exceed the maximum allowable 640 calories for this meal.

<u>Diet Tip of the Day:</u> Know your **daily caloric allowance** whether you are trying to maintain your weight or are on a reducing diet. (See "***Weight Control - U.S. Edition***" a NoPaperPress eBook where you can determine your daily caloric allowance using unique Weight Maintenance tables.)

Day 80 - Recipe

<u>Vegetable Chili</u>

1	tablespoon olive oil
2	medium carrots, cut into ½-inch pieces
2	medium parsnips, cut into ½-inch pieces
1	medium onion, chopped
2	cans (15-ounces each) red kidney beans, drained
4	teaspoons chili powder
1	can (28-ounce) whole tomatoes in juice
¼	cup fresh cilantro leaves, chopped

In saucepot, heat olive oil on medium-high. Add carrots, parsnips, chopped onion, and cook 6 to 8 minutes or until all vegetables are tender and beginning to brown, stirring occasionally.

Meanwhile, on large plate, mash 1 cup drained beans. Stir chili powder into vegetables in saucepot; cook 1 minute, stirring. Add canned tomatoes with their juice, whole and mashed beans, and 2 cups water. Heat to boiling on high, breaking up tomatoes with spoon. Reduce heat to medium and cook, uncovered for 10 minutes, stirring occasionally. Finally, stir in cilantro and serve.

<u>**Serves 4**</u>. 360 Calories per serving

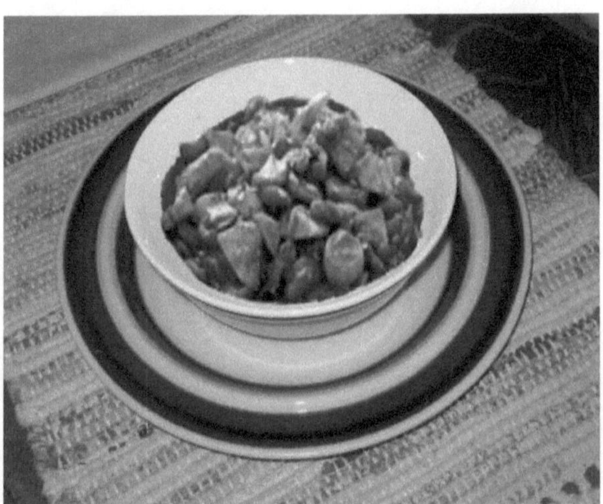

<u>**Diet Tip of the Day:**</u> **Carbohydrates** provide your body with its basic fuel, the energy your cells need to survive, as well as essential vitamins and minerals, fiber, and other beneficial compounds that promote good health.

Day 81 - Recipe

<u>Frozen-Meat Dinner</u>

No recipe today. No cooking today. It's your day off! To find a frozen meat dinner entrée please go to Appendix A (page 198) which lists approximately 150 frozen dinners manufactured by Healthy Choice, Lean Cuisine and Smart Ones.

Note that if you do not use all of the **300 Calories allocated for the Day 21 frozen dinner**, use the excess calories anyway you wish. Splurge on extra dessert or save the calories for another day.

Please read the important **Frozen-Food Safety Warning** in Appendix B on page 204.

<u>**Diet Tip of the Day:**</u> Keep low-calorie **lean sandwich fixings on hand** (whole-wheat bread, sliced turkey, reduced-fat cheese, lettuce, tomatoes and mustard).

Chicken Salad

    4 skinless, boneless chicken breast halves (½ lb total)
    1 cup carrots, sliced
    1 cup red bell peppers, sliced
    4 green onions, diced
    1 cup edamame beans, cooked and shelled
    1 cup chow mien noodles
    2 hearts romaine lettuce
    4 cups mesclun mix or spring mix

Salad dressing: In a jar with a tight-fitting lid combine 2 tsp garlic powder, 1 tsp dried parsley, 1 tsp dried basil, 1 tsp honey, 2 tsp soy sauce, 4 tsp sesame oil, 2 tsp Sriracha (hot sauce – optional), 4 tsp Dijon mustard, 4 tbsp olive oil, 4 tbsp rice wine vinegar and a dash of black pepper. Shake well and set aside.

Grill chicken breast halves and then cut them into small pieces.

In a bowl, combine romaine lettuce, mesclun mix lettuces (or spring mix), carrots, red bell pepper, green onions and edamame. Add the dressing and toss. Add chow mien noodles and chicken and toss again.
Serves 4. 440 Calories per serving

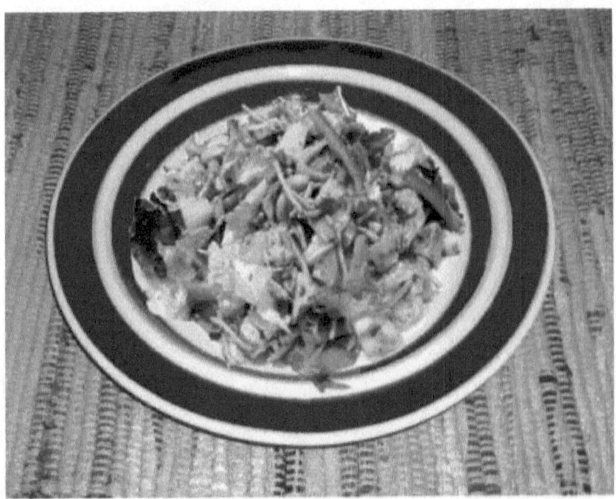

Diet Tip of the Day: Do not eat foods containing partially-hydrogenated vegetable oil because they are high in **trans fats**. This includes commercially prepared baked goods, snack foods, and processed foods, including most fast foods.

<u>Hearty Lentil Stew</u>

½ cup chopped onion
2   garlic cloves, minced
1   tablespoon vegetable oil
1   cup lentils, rinsed
4   tsp vegetable or chicken bouillon granules
3   tsp Worcestershire sauce
1   bay leaf
1   cup chopped carrots
14.5-ounce can diced tomatoes with liquid
10-oz package frozen chopped spinach, thawed
1   Tbsp red wine vinegar

In a large saucepan, sauté onion and garlic in oil until tender. Add 5 cups of water, lentils, bouillon, Worcestershire sauce, ½ teaspoon salt, ¼ teaspoon black pepper and the bay leaf. Bring to a boil. Reduce heat; cover and simmer for 20 minutes.

Add the carrots, tomatoes and spinach; return to a boil. Reduce heat; cover and simmer additional 15 to 20 minutes, or until lentils are tender. Stir in vinegar and serve.

<u>Serves 4</u>. 260 Calories per serving

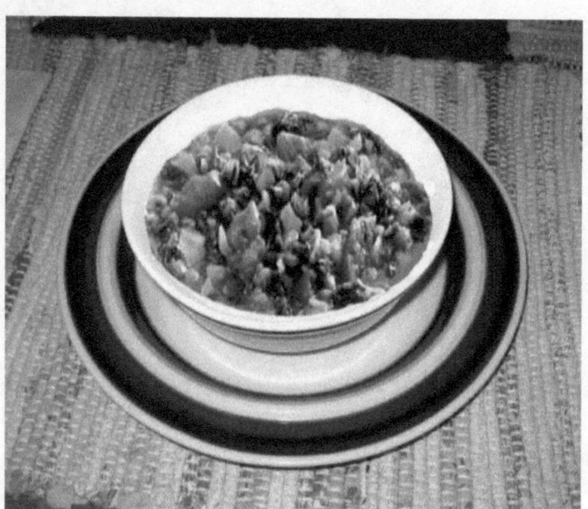

<u>Diet Tip of the Day:</u> Monounsaturated fats "**good fats**" are derived from plant sources, such as vegetable oils, nuts, and seeds. This type of fat is found in high concentrations in canola, olive and peanut oils.

<u>Turkey Burger</u>

- 1¼ pounds ground turkey
- 1   tablespoon Worcestershire sauce
- 1   tablespoon chipotle mustard
- 1   tablespoon olive oil for brushing
- 4   seeded hamburger rolls

Lightly mix together the ground turkey, Worcestershire sauce, mustard, salt and black pepper. Form into 4 patties and brush each side lightly with olive oil.

Heat grill to medium-high. Place patties on grill and cook for 3 to 4 minutes each side for medium-well done. Salt and pepper to taste.

<u>Serves 4</u>. 355 Calories per serving (turkey burger only)

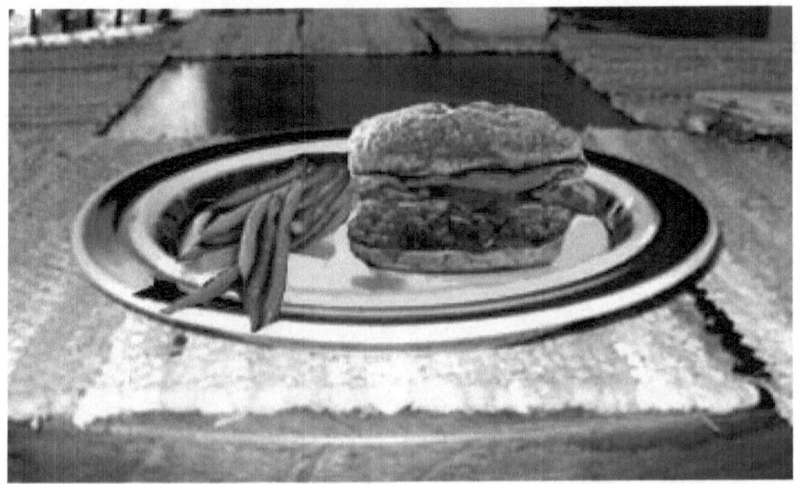

<u>Diet Tip of the Day:</u> Consistently **choose healthy foods**, avoid harmful foods and large portions and exercise regularly. Nothing else will control your weight over the long haul.

Day 85 - Recipe

<u>Carrie's Low-Cal Meat Loaf</u>

½ pound ground white meat turkey
½ pound ground beef (about 90% lean)
1 large egg
½ cup skim milk
¼ cup bread crumbs
¼ cup ketchup
¼ cup chopped carrots
¼ cup chopped onion

In a medium bowl, combine all ingredients. Add salt and pepper to taste. Mix until blended and form into a loaf. Place loaf into oven preheated to 350 °F. Bake until an instant-read thermometer inserted in the center of the loaf reads 160 °F. This should take about one hour.

Shown below is meat loaf, acorn squash (baked with 1 teaspoon of maple syrup). Also shown is steamed spinach drizzled with extra-virgin olive oil. <u>Serves 5</u>. About 290 Calories per serving (for meat loaf only). Note that half a serving of left over meat loaf is to be eaten for lunch on Day 87.

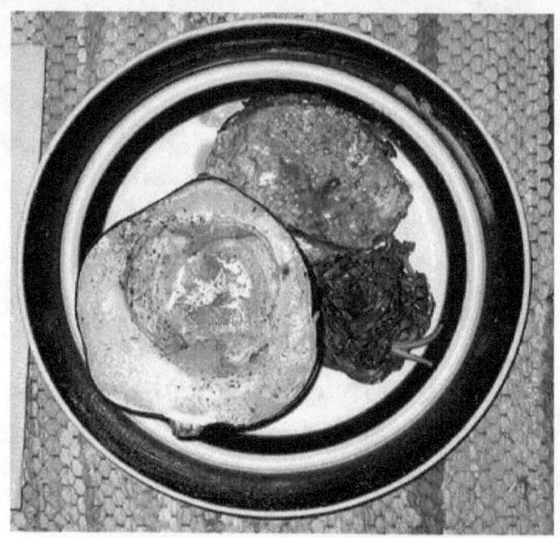

<u>Diet Tip of the Day</u>: Your **body weight fluctuates** two to three pounds daily. Your body weight is lowest before breakfast and highest in the evening before you retire.

Day 86 - Recipe

<u>Tuna & Bean Salad</u>

1	tuna steak, about 2 inches thick (14 ounces)
2	tablespoons extra-virgin olive oil
1	tablespoon lemon juice
1	garlic clove, crushed
1	tablespoon Dijon mustard
1	15-ounce can cannellini beans, drained
1	small red onion, thinly sliced
2	red peppers, seeded and thinly sliced
½	cucumber, halved lengthwise and thinly sliced
6	cups watercress

Heat a ridged grill pan coated with cooking spray over medium-high heat. Season tuna steak on both sides with coarsely ground black pepper. Cook the tuna 4 minutes on each side - the outside should be browned and the center light pink. Be careful not to overcook. Remove from the pan and set aside.

Mix together the oil, lemon juice, garlic, and mustard in a salad bowl. Season with salt and pepper to taste. Add the cannellini beans, onion, peppers, cucumber and watercress. Toss gently to mix. Cut tuna into ½-inch thick slices. Arrange on top of salad and serve with lemon wedges.
<u>Serves 4</u>. 355 Calories per serving

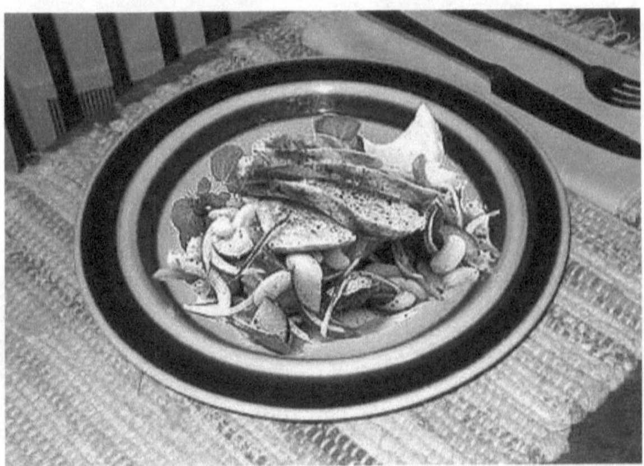

<u>Diet Tip of the Day:</u> In the United States, for a food to be labeled "**whole grain**" it must contain more than 51 percent whole grain by weight.

Day 87 - Recipe

Pasta and Veggies

- ¾ pound penne pasta
- 2 cups broccoli florets
- 1 red bell pepper, sliced
- 1 carrot, cut to 1-inch sticks
- ½ cup frozen green peas & ½ cup frozen sweet corn
- 1 small onion, chopped
- 1 tablespoon minced garlic
- 3 tablespoons olive oil
- 1 teaspoon fresh basil, chopped

Cook penne pasta per package directions. Drain and place pasta in a bowl. Pre-cook the carrot and broccoli florets.

In a large heavy skillet, heat the olive oil and sauté onion and garlic until lightly golden. Add vegetables and sauté until the peppers are soft. Combine sautéed vegetables in the bowl with the pasta. Toss well. Garnish with chopped basil, season to taste, and top with freshly grated Parmesan cheese. **Serves 4**. 460 Calories per serving

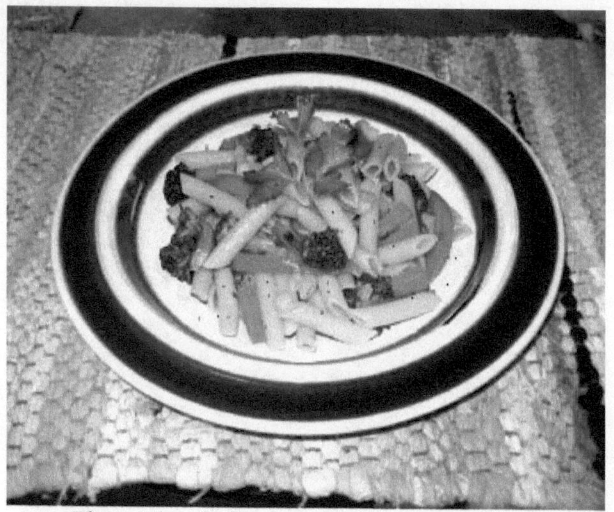

Photo taken before grated cheese was added.

Diet Tip of the Day: When possible, **select fresh and natural foods** and whole-grain products. Avoid chemical preservatives and additives, artificial and imitation foods, refined and processed foods, and foods that are comprised of "nutritionally-empty calories."

<u>Frozen Chicken Dinner</u>

No recipe today. No cooking today. It's your day off! To find a frozen chicken dinner entrée please go to Appendix A (page 198) which lists approximately 150 frozen dinners manufactured by Healthy Choice, Lean Cuisine and Smart Ones.

Note that if you do not use all of the **300 Calories allocated for the Day 56 frozen dinner**, use the excess calories anyway you wish. Splurge on extra dessert or save the calories for another day.

Please read the important **Frozen-Food Safety Warning** in Appendix B on page 204.

<u>**Diet Tip of the Day:**</u> Understand that the only **sure way to slim down for keeps** is to eat less and exercise more. There are no safe short cuts or miracle methods for taking off weight.

Fish Stew

1	pound shrimp, peeled and de-veined
¾	pound skinless flounder fillet, cut into strips
1	pound new baby potatoes, halved
2	peppers (red and yellow) sliced into strips
1	onion, halved and sliced
4	ounces white wine
2	cups vegetable stock
2	cloves garlic, crushed
1	small bunch basil, shredded
1½	tablespoons olive oil

In a large pot, sauté garlic, onion and peppers in olive oil until they are completely softened. Stir in wine, vegetable stock and potatoes. Simmer until potatoes are tender.

Add the shrimp and flounder and cook for additional 4 minutes. Stir in basil and serve.

Serves 4. 300 Calories per serving

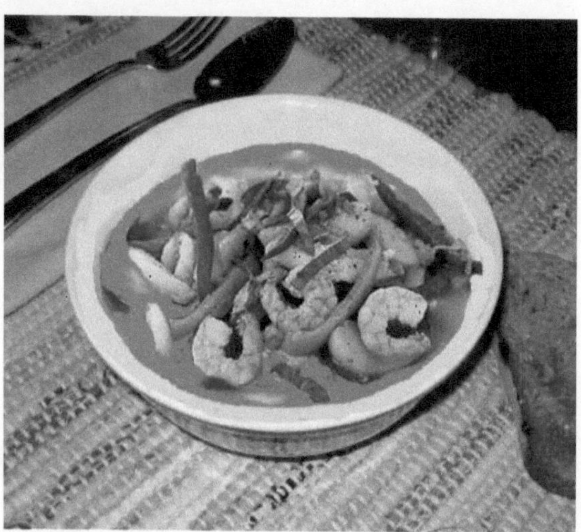

Diet Tip of the Day: All **fish** are relatively low-calorie foods and are good sources of protein and fat-soluble vitamins A and D.

<u>Veal with Mushrooms & Tomato</u>

- ½ pound spaghetti
- ¾ pound veal cutlets
- 8 ounces sliced mushrooms
- 2 tablespoon olive oil, divided
- 2 tablespoons flour
- 3 green onions, small, sliced
- ½ cup chicken broth
- 14.5-ounce can diced tomatoes

Pound veal to about ¼-inch thickness. Rinse, pat dry and cut into 2-inch pieces. Heat 1 tablespoon olive oil in large nonstick skillet over medium heat. Add mushrooms and cook, stirring, until lightly browned. Remove and set aside.

Season veal with salt and pepper and coat lightly with flour. Add remaining olive oil to skillet and cook veal over medium heat for about 2 minutes on each side, or until browned. Add the green onions and cook for 1 minute longer. Add chicken broth and cook, uncovered, for 5 minutes. Add tomatoes; cover and simmer for 3 to 5 minutes. Serve over spaghetti cooked per package directions.

<u>Serves 4</u>. 520 Calories per serving (includes spaghetti)

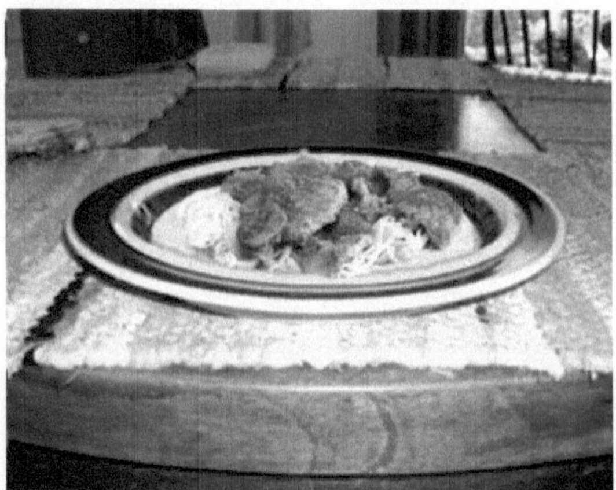

<u>Diet Tip of the Day:</u> Successful weight loss and subsequent weight maintenance **requires knowledge, desire and discipline**. Avoid the latest fad diets. Instead, take the time to develop a true understanding of weight control and then change your eating and activity habits accordingly.

Appendix A
Frozen Entrees

Appendix D lists three popular brands of frozen entrées: Healthy Choice, Lean Cuisine and Smart Ones. Note that each brand is color coded. The listing is further divided by entrée type: Poultry entrées, Meat entrées, Seafood entrées, Pasta entrées, Pizza and Other entrées. The entire table is arranged from the lowest to highest in calories. Note that the listed frozen entrées were available in most super markets as of 07/14/2020.

Entrée Type	Name	Brand	Calories
Poultry	Tomato Basil Chicken & Spinach	Smart Ones	160
Meat	Steak Portobella	Lean Cuisine	160
Meat	Asian Style Beef & Broccoli	Smart Ones	~~160~~ 170
Poultry	Herb Roasted Chicken	Lean Cuisine	170
Poultry	Slow Roasted Turkey Breast	Smart Ones	170
Poultry	Grilled Chicken Marsala	Healthy Choice	180
Poultry	Creamy Basil Chicken w Broccoli	Smart Ones	~~180~~ 170
Poultry	Garlic Chicken Rolls	Lean Cuisine	180
Meat	Beef Merlot	Healthy Choice	180
Meat	Homestyle Beef Pot Roast	Smart Ones	180
Poultry	Roasted Turkey & Vegetables	Lean Cuisine	190
Poultry	Chicken & Broccoli Alfredo	Healthy Choice	190
Poultry	Chicken & Vegetable Stir Fry	Healthy Choice	190
Other	Broccoli & Cheddar Roast Potato	Smart Ones	190
Poultry	Home Style Chicken & Potatoes	Healthy Choice	200
Poultry	Crustless Chicken Pot Pie	Smart Ones	~~200~~ 190
Poultry	Buffalo Style Chicken	Lean Cuisine	~~200~~ 190
Pasta	Angel Hair Marinara	Smart Ones	200
Poultry	Salisbury Steak	Smart Ones	200

Meat	Roast Beef & Mashed Potatoes	Smart Ones	~~220~~ 200
Pasta	Primavera Pasta	Smart Ones	210
Poultry	Honey Balsamic Chicken	Healthy Choice	210
Pasta	Ravioli Florentine	Smart Ones	210
Poultry	Cajun Style Chicken & Shrimp	Healthy Choice	220
Pasta	Cheese Ravioli Mushroom Sauce	Smart Ones	230
Poultry	Ranchero Chicken Wrap	Smart Ones	230
Poultry	Lemon Herb Chicken Picante	Smart Ones	230
Pasta	Cheese Ravioli Mushroom Sauce	Smart Ones	230
Meat	Meat Loaf with Mashed Potatoes	Lean Cuisine	~~230~~ 240
Seafood	Shrimp Alfredo	Lean Cuisine	~~230~~ 240
Poultry	Chicken Margherita	Smart Ones	~~220~~ 240
Poultry	Grilled Chicken Caesar	Lean Cuisine	240
Poultry	Honey Glazed Turkey & Potatoes	Healthy Choice	240
Pasta	Spicy Penne Arrabbiata	Lean Cuisine	240
Pasta	Four Cheese Cannelloni	Lean Cuisine	~~240~~ 250
Poultry	Creamy Basil Chicken w Tortellini	Lean Cuisine	~~240~~ 250
Pasta	Cheese Ravioli	Lean Cuisine	250
Pasta	Vermont Cheddar Mac & Cheese	Lean Cuisine	250
Pasta	Fettuccini Alfredo	Smart Ones	250
Poultry	Oriental Chicken	Smart Ones	250
Poultry	Fiesta Grilled Chicken	Lean Cuisine	250
Pasta	Chicken Linguini Red Pepper	Healthy Choice	250
Poultry	Golden Roasted Turkey Breast	Healthy Choice	250
Poultry	Chicken Mesquite	Smart Ones	250
Poultry	Chicken Oriental	Smart Ones	250
Poultry	Orange Sesame Chicken	Smart Ones	250
Poultry	Baked Chicken	Lean Cuisine	~~250~~ 260
Poultry	Teriyaki Chicken & Vegetables	Smart Ones	~~250~~ 260

Seafood	Tuna Noodle Casserole	Smart Ones	~~250~~ 270
Pasta	Spaghetti with Meatballs	Lean Cuisine	260
Poultry	Creamy Chicken & Noodles	Healthy Choice	260
Meat	Barbecue Steak w Red Potatoes	Healthy Choice	260
Pasta	Tortellini Primavera Parmesan	Healthy Choice	260
Pasta	Sesame Noodles with Vegetables	Smart Ones	~~260~~ 280
Pasta	Creamy Rigatoni w Chicken	Smart Ones	260
Pasta	Macaroni & Cheese	Smart Ones	260
Pasta	Butternut Squash Ravioli	Lean Cuisine	260
Other	Santa Fe Rice & Beans	Smart Ones	260
Other	Coconut Chickpea Curry	Lean Cuisine	260
Poultry	Glazed Turkey Tenderloins	Lean Cuisine	270
Poultry	Kung Pao Chicken	Healthy Choice	270
Poultry	Chicken Margherita w Balsamic	Healthy Choice	270
Poultry	Chicken Strips & Sweet Potatoes	Smart Ones	270
Pasta	Spaghetti with Meat Sauce	Smart Ones	~~270~~ 280
Meat	Salisbury Steak with Mac & Cheese	Lean Cuisine	~~270~~ 290
Pasta	Penne Rosa	Lean Cuisine	270
Poultry	Turkey Breast & Stuffing	Smart Ones	~~270~~ 280
Pasta	Classic Macaroni & Beef	Lean Cuisine	270
Pasta	Mushroom Mezzaluna Ravioli	Lean Cuisine	270
Pasta	Pasta with Swedish Meatballs	Smart Ones	~~280~~ 290
Other	Asian Pot Stickers	Lean Cuisine	280
Poultry	Sesame Stir Fry with Chicken	Lean Cuisine	280
Poultry	Roasted Turkey Breast	Lean Cuisine	~~280~~ 290
Poultry	Apple Cranberry Chicken	Lean Cuisine	280
Poultry	Chicken Fettuccini Alfredo	Healthy Choice	280
Poultry	Grilled Chicken Marinara	Healthy Choice	280
Poultry	Sweet & Spicy Orange Chicken	Healthy Choice	280

Category	Meal	Brand	Calories
Poultry	Chicken Parmesan	Smart Ones	280
Poultry	Turkey Breast with Stuffing	Smart Ones	280
Meat	Beef & Broccoli	Healthy Choice	280
Meat	Meatball Marinara	Healthy Choice	280
Meat	Beef Teriyaki	Healthy Choice	280
Pasta	Spinach Artichoke Ravioli	Lean Cuisine	280
Other	Vegetable Fried Rice	Smart Ones	280
Pasta	Spinach Artichoke Ravioli	Lean Cuisine	280
Pasta	Linguini with Ricotta & Spinach	Lean Cuisine	280
Poultry	Chicken Fettuccini	Lean Cuisine	~~290~~ 280
Pasta	Spaghetti & Meatballs	Healthy Choice	280
Pasta	Spaghetti with Meat Sauce	Smart Ones	280
Other	Vegetable Fried Rice	Smart Ones	280
Other	Asian Pot Stickers	Lean Cuisine	280
Poultry	Chicken with Almonds	Lean Cuisine	290
Poultry	Chicken with Peanut Sauce	Lean Cuisine	290
Seafood	Shrimp & Angel Hair Pasta	Lean Cuisine	~~280~~ 290
Poultry	Grilled Chicken Pesto w Veggies	Healthy Choice	290
Poultry	General Tso's Spicy Chicken	Healthy Choice	290
Poultry	Pineapple Chicken	Healthy Choice	290
Poultry	Chicken Enchiladas Suiza	Smart Ones	290
Meat	Swedish Meatballs	Lean Cuisine	290
Seafood	Lemon Pepper Fish	Healthy Choice	290
Pasta	Pasta with Swedish Meatballs	Smart Ones	290
Other	Santa Fe Rice & Beans	Smart Ones	290
Pizza	Thin Crust Cheese Pizza	Smart Ones	290
Seafood	Parmesan Crusted Fish	Lean Cuisine	~~290~~ 300
Pasta	Santa Fe-Style Rice & Beans	Lean Cuisine	~~280~~ 300
Poultry	Roasted Turkey & Vegetables	Lean Cuisine	~~290~~ 300

Poultry	Sweet & Sour Chicken	Lean Cuisine	300
Poultry	Crustless Chicken Pot Pie	Healthy Choice	300
Poultry	Sweet Sesame Chicken	Healthy Choice	300
Poultry	Chicken Fettuccini	Smart Ones	300
Poultry	General Tso's Chicken	Smart Ones	300
Meat	Classic Meat Loaf	Healthy Choice	300
Seafood	Tortilla Crusted Fish	Lean Cuisine	~~300~~ 310
Pasta	Tuscan-Style Vegetable Lasagna	Lean Cuisine	~~300~~ 310
Pasta	Tortellini with Red Pepper Sauce	Lean Cuisine	300
Pasta	Broccoli Cheddar Rotini	Lean Cuisine	300
Pasta	Three Cheese Ziti Marinara	Smart Ones	300
Pasta	Lasagna Florentine	Smart Ones	~~310~~ 300
Seafood	Tortilla Crusted Fish	Lean Cuisine	~~300~~ 310
Pasta	Tuscan-Style Vegetable Lasagna	Lean Cuisine	~~300~~ 310
Poultry	Chicken Fried Rice	Lean Cuisine	~~300~~ 310
Poultry	Orange Chicken	Lean Cuisine	310
Poultry	Chicken Tikka Masala	Lean Cuisine	310
Poultry	Chicken Strips & Fries	Smart Ones	310
Poultry	Chicken Teriyaki	Lean Cuisine	310
Pizza	Thin Crust Pepperoni Pizza	Smart Ones	310
Pasta	Three Cheese Macaroni	Smart Ones	310
Pizza	French Bread Pepperoni Pizza	Lean Cuisine	310
Poultry	Chicken Spinach Mushroom Panini	Lean Cuisine	~~350~~ 310
Other	Spicy Beef & Bean Enchilada	Lean Cuisine	310
Poultry	Chicken Fried Rice	Healthy Choice	320
Meat	Sweet & Spicy Korean Beef	Lean Cuisine	320
Pizza	Farmers Market Pizza	Lean Cuisine	320
Pizza	Margherita Pizza	Lean Cuisine	320
Poultry	Chicken Carbonara	Lean Cuisine	330

Poultry	Mango Chicken w Coconut Rice	Lean Cuisine	330
Poultry	Country Fried Chicken	Healthy Choice	330
Other	Cheese & Fire-Roasted Tamale	Lean Cuisine	330
Poultry	Chicken Club Panini	Lean Cuisine	~~350~~ 340
Meat	Philly Style Steak & Cheese Panini	Lean Cuisine	~~330~~ 350
Poultry	Chicken Parmigiana	Healthy Choice	360
Poultry	Chicken Pecan	Lean Cuisine	~~320~~ 370
Poultry	Sweet & Sour Chicken	Healthy Choice	390
Pizza	Supreme Pizza	Lean Cuisine	~~330~~ 390

Appendix B
Frozen Food Safety

Increasingly, food giants like ConAgra, Nestlé and others that supply Americans with processed foods concede that they cannot ensure the safety of their food products. Frozen foods pose a particularly serious safety problem because unsuspecting consumers buy frozen foods for their convenience and incorrectly believe that cooking frozen foods is a matter of taste – not safety. Still the food industry says that extensive outbreaks of food-borne illness are rare, even though it is well-known that most of the millions of cases of food-borne illness every year go unreported or are not traced to the source. For example, each year approximately 40,000 cases of salmonella poisoning are reported in the United States – but perhaps as many as one million cases go unreported. (Salmonella is a type of bacteria most often found in poultry, eggs, unprocessed milk, meat and water.)   Recently salmonella pathogens in some frozen meals have sickened thousands of people.

How could this happen? First, the supply chain for ingredients in processed foods – from flour to fruits and vegetables to flavorings – is becoming more complex and global in the drive to keep food costs down. As a result, government and industry officials concede that almost every food ingredient is now a potential carrier of pathogens. A further complication is that a large number of food companies subcontract processing work to save money and don't require suppliers to test for pathogens. In fact, companies often don't even know who is supplying their ingredients.

In addition, many frozen-food manufacturers have stopped cooking their products at high temperatures, a tactic they call the "kill step," which is intended to eliminate any lingering microbes. Frequently this process step turns some of the frozen food ingredients into mush. So, instead the "kill step" has been shifted to consumers. For example, ConAgra has added food safety instructions to its frozen meals, including the Healthy Choice brand. A typical "frozen-food safety" instruction offers this guidance: "Internal temperature needs to reach 165°F as measured by a food thermometer in several spots."

General Mills, now advises consumers to avoid microwaves altogether and cook their frozen pizzas only in a conventional oven. To be safe, always cook frozen foods so the internal temperature reaches 165°F.

Appendix C
Soup Selections

The following lists **canned** soup selections. See the important note at the end of list. The soup listed below were available in supermarkets as of 06/25/2020.

	<u>Soup</u>	Calories
1	Progresso Chicken and Wild Rice	80
2	Progresso Hearty Chicken and Rotini	90
3	Progresso Garden Vegetable	90
4	Progresso Minestrone	110
5	Progresso Chickarina	110
6	Progresso Italian Wedding	120
7	Progresso Split Pea	130
8	Progresso Tuscan-Style White Bean	130
9	Progresso Lentil	140
10	Progresso Tomato Basil	150
11	Progresso Macaroni & Bean	160
12	Progresso Hearty Penne	160
13	Progresso Three Cheese Tortellini	170

* **Important:** When the Daily Meal Plan menu specifies soup, have <u>only one serving</u> (8 oz) unless stated otherwise.

To improve the taste of canned soup, add a teaspoon of grated cheese before heating the soup in a microwave oven. After heating, add ½ teaspoon of olive oil. Stir and serve. These additions enhance the taste, and total about 30 Calories which should be added to the soup calories shown in the table above.

NoPaperPress eBooks and Paperbacks

100-Day Super Diet-1200 Cal*
100-Day Super Diet-1500 Cal*
100-Day No-Cooking Diet-1200 Cal*
100-Day No-Cooking Diet-1500 Cal*
90-Day Smart Diet-1200 Cal*
90-Day Smart Diet-1500 Cal*
90-Day No-Cooking Diet - 1200 Cal*
90-Day No-Cooking Diet - 1500 Cal*
90-Day Perfect Diet - 1200 Cal*
90-Day Perfect Diet - 1500 Cal*
60-Day Perfect Diet-1200 Cal*
60-Day Perfect Diet-1500 Cal*
50-Day Flex Diet-1200 Cal*
50-Day Flex Diet-1500 Cal*
30-Day Quick Diet - Women*
30-Day Quick Diet for Men*
30-Day No-Cooking Diet*
30-Day Diet for Women - Metric*
30-Day Diet for Men - Metric*
25 Day Easy Diet-1200 Cal*
25 Day Easy Diet-1500 Cal*
25-Day No-Cooking Diet
10-Day Express Diet
10-Day No-Cooking Diet*
7-Day Diet for Women*
7-Day Diet for Men*
7-Day No-Cooking Diets*
90-Day Gluten-Free Diet-1200 Cal*
90-Day Gluten-Free Diet-1500 Cal*
30-Day Gluten-Free Quick Diet*
30-Day Gluten-Free No-Cooking Diet*
7-Day Diet for Women - Metric*
7-Day Diet for Men - Metric
7-Day Gluten-Free Express Diet*
7-Day Gluten-Free No-Cooking Diet*
90-Day Vegetarian Diet-1200 Cal*
90-Day Vegetarian Diet-1500 Cal*
30-Day Vegetarian Diet*
7-Day Vegetarian Diet*
Weight Loss for Women*
Weight Loss for Women - Metric
Weight Loss for Women - UK
Weight Loss for Men*
Maximum Weight Loss - 1200 Cal*
Maximum Weight Loss - 1500 Cal*

Weight Loss for Men - Metric*
Maximum Weight Loss- 1200 Cal*
Maximum Weight Loss- 1500 Cal*
Weight Control - U.S. Edition*
Weight Control - Metric. Edition
Professional Weight Control Women - U.S.
Professional Weight Control Women - Metric
Professional Weight Control Men - U.S.
Professional Weight Control Men - Metric
Weight Maintenance - U.S. Ed*
Weight Maintenance - Metric. Ed*
Weight Maintenance - UK Ed
Weight Loss for Senior Men*
Weight Loss for Senior Women*
Eat Smart - U.S. Edition*
Eat Smart - Metric Edition
30-Day Mediterranean Diet
Exercise Smart - U.S. Edition*
Exercise Smart - Metric Edition
Exercise Smart - UK Edition*
Total Fitness - U.S. Edition
Total Fitness - Metric Edition
Total Fitness - UK Edition
Total Fitness for Women-U.S. Ed*
Total Fitness for Women - Metric
Total Fitness for Women - UK Ed
Total Fitness for Men - U.S. Ed*
Total Fitness for Men- Metric Ed*
Total Fitness for Men - UK Ed
Senior Fitness - U.S. Edition*
Senior Fitness - Metric Edition*
Senior Fitness - UK Edition*
Computer Diet - U.S. Edition*
Computer Diet - Metric Ed*
Reliable Weight Loss - U.S. Ed
101 Weight Loss Tips*
101 Healthy Eating Tips*
101 Lifelong Fitness Tips*
101 Weight Maintenance Tips
101 Weight Loss Recipes
101 GF Weight Loss Recipes
101 Veggie Weight Loss Recipes*
30-Day Mediterranean Diet*
90-Day Mediterranean Diet - 1200 Cal*
90-Day Mediterranean Diet - 1500 Cal*

* These titles are available as both ebooks and paperbacks. Our ebooks are sold by Amazon, Apple, Google, Barnes & Noble and Kobo, but our paperbacks are only sold by Amazon.

Disclaimer

This book offers general meal planning, nutrition and weight control information. It is not a medical manual and the author does not claim to be medically qualified. The material in this book is not intended to be a substitute for medical counseling. Everyone should have a medical checkup before beginning a weight loss program. Moreover, the physician conducting the medical exam should be made aware of and should approve the specific weight control program planned. Additionally, while the author and publisher have made every effort to ensure the accuracy of the information in this book, they make no representations or warranties regarding its accuracy or completeness. Further, neither the author nor publisher assume liability for any medical problems that might result from applying the methods in this book, or for any loss of profit, or any other commercial damages, including but not limited to special, incidental, consequential or other damages, and any such liability is hereby expressly disclaimed.